# ALLERGY?
# THINK
# ABOUT FOOD

'One of the major problems with many additives is that they are known to cause allergies. If you do have one which you cannot trace, it would be worth investing in a paperback called Allergy? Think About Food.'
**Daily Telegraph**

'A diary is the best weapon for a food detective says Susan Lewis. If you think your child is allergic to some sort of food, list everything they can eat and drink and how they feel.'
**News of the World**

'The book should encourage allergy sufferers to think more inquisitively about food without destroying the pleasure.'
**House & Garden**

'If you want to find out whether food or drink is the cause of your – your child's – allergy, Susan Lewis has written a helpful, easy-to-understand book.'
**Weekend**

# ALLERGY?
# THINK
# ABOUT FOOD

'Susan Lewis has written an immensely readable book on how avoidance of certain foods can bring about relief of many conditions. . . . it is a must for everyone's bookcase, and sensibly priced.'
**The Hyperactive Children's Support Group Journal**

'In her practical, very readable book she is at pains to point out that just because one food causes similar symptoms in somebody else it does not necessarily account for your own.'
**Sunday Times**

'. . . the book is packed with useful practical information and could be recommended to people who have just realised that their food might be affecting them . . .'
**Society of Environmental Therapy**

'Unconverted readers of the book will be made to stop and think and the converted will find many useful tips in their search for a symptom free existence.'
**Midwife, Health Visitor and Community Nurse**

# ALLERGY?
# THINK
# ABOUT FOOD

# ALLERGY?
# THINK
# ABOUT FOOD

'One book which seems to stand out is Allergy? Think About Food. It is written in an easy-to-read, easy to understand style and gives a comprehensive guide to foods, what they contain and the laws on labelling in the UK.'
**Asthma News, The Asthma Society**

'Anyone who wants to find out if they or their children have an allergy to a food or drink would find this a useful book.'
**Nursing Mirror**

'. . . the layman will also find a new publication by Susan Lewis, called Allergy? Think About Food, a great help. This is a logical and very down-to-earth guide to the subject.'
**National Eczema Society Magazine**

# ALLERGY?
# THINK
# ABOUT FOOD

**Allergy? Think About Food was chosen by the British Council to be exhibited on its stand at the Frankfurt Book Fair in October 1985 and the Copenhagen Book Fair in November 1985.**

'I received the copy of Allergy? Think About Food which to my mind is the best on the market of its kind. Would you kindly let me have two more copies which I want to pass on to friends.'
**Mrs M. R. Oxford**

'I enjoyed your book very much and am enjoying even more eating a purer diet as a result . . . Thank you anyway for a most informative book.
**Mrs P. S. D. London**

'I think it is a very good book – especially as it is so thorough and so practical and easy to understand.'
**Mrs E. B. Inverness**

'Your book Allergy? Think About Food has been recommended to me as the best one about this matter.'
**Mrs E. J. London**

This book will help you discover whether food or drink is the cause of your, or your child's allergy. It will help you pinpoint the 'safe' foods which can be eaten as well as those causing trouble and can easily be used by both adults and children.

With the help of real life examples, Susan Lewis documents how ordinary men and women found that sometimes serious and disabling conditions could be cured 'miraculously'. Rashes, wheezing, headaches, hyperactivity, bedwetting, stomach upsets, aches and pains, and even mental illness disappeared once a food or drink was eliminated.

# ALLERGY?
# THINK
# ABOUT FOOD

## Susan Lewis

**WISEBUY PUBLICATIONS**

*First published 1984*
*Second edition 1986*

*Copyright © 1984, 1986 Wisebuy Publications*

Published in the Dutch language as *Voeding En
Allergie* by Uitgeverij Elmar, Netherlands.

**British Library Cataloguing in Publication Data**
Lewis, Susan
  Allergy? Think About Food – 2nd ed.
  1. Food allergy
  I. Title
  616.97′5   RC596

  ISBN 0-9509751-1-7

*Printed in Great Britain by
Hunt Barnard Printing Ltd., Aylesbury, Bucks.*

# Contents

# Acknowledgements

The examples of food allergy quoted in this book come from 230 letters. My thanks go to those who took the trouble to write about their experiences. I hope their stories will help others think about the possible connection between their health and what they eat.

Two doctors, a hospital dietician, a food technologist, a lawyer and a school librarian read through the final draft of this book and made many useful comments and suggestions. Thank you (in alphabetical order) Liz Bark-Jones, Ginny Saffron, Norma Silverton, Isobel Skypala, David Solomons and Richard Stone.

I would like to thank the personnel at the Ministry of Agriculture, Fisheries and Food; and David Smith and Jack Weiner for looking through various draft chapters. My gratitude also goes to the organisations and manufacturers mentioned in this book who checked their sections for accuracy.

Finally my thanks go to my husband, David, who edited the book and gave me the encouragement I needed to write it and my two children, especially Duncan, without whom this book would never have been written.

# Preface to second edition

Significant changes have taken place to the benefit of food allergy sufferers since the first edition of this book. In July 1986 new Food Labelling Regulations came into effect enabling customers to identify far more easily those potentially dangerous additives used in processed products. Details of the new regulations are given in Chapter 4.

The new labelling laws together with the public's demand for less use of food additives have started a minor revolution within the food industry. Manufacturers are beginning to review the amount of additives added to their products and the necessity for them. Those food chains making a change are described in Chapter 8.

This second edition of Allergy? Think About Food includes even more details of food additives thought to cause trouble (see Chapter 10) and a greatly expanded list of permitted additives and their code numbers explaining what they are and where they are used. These are given in Appendix 2.

Throughout the book new information about the food and drink you buy has been included plus hints and thoughts which will help you discover any link between your allergy and its cause. It tells you more about ˜bread and flour, gives more details of natural chemicals found in food such as salicylates and tyramine, explains what to do about inaccurate labelling and lists extra useful names and addresses of organisations able to help you.

Toothpaste, although not a food, is daily absorbed into the body and actually swallowed by many children. Legally toothpaste ingredients do not have to be disclosed and these ingredients are revealed in Chapter 12.

*Susan Lewis*

# 1

# Food is good for you . . .
## . . . but not always

In the spring of 1983, two national newspapers published a letter from me asking readers 'if they had discovered any foods or additives to which they or their children were allergic, what the effects were and how they had managed to pinpoint the cause.' I received 266 replies of which 230 convincingly wrote that a single food, several foods, or their ingredients were the cause of symptoms.

Sixty-one were sufferers with breathing difficulties: asthma, hayfever or cold-like symptoms such as sneezing, coughing, runny or blocked noses. Seventy-three suffered from skin complaints like eczema, urticaria (nettlerash, red raised bumps), other rashes and swellings. And twenty-nine got headaches or migraine. Twenty-eight letters were from parents of children suffering from hyperactivity (unusual behaviour) and another six concerned children with a bed-wetting problem. Nineteen people mentioned stomach complaints such as indigestion, cramp, sickness and diarrhoea. Six suffered from aches and pains. Three writers suffered from depression and nightmares. Two letters described fits and convulsions and three mentioned shaking or fainting.

The severity of the symptoms varied enormously from the relatively unimportant (except to the sufferer) to those which needed medical or even hospital treatment. The foods or additives which caused the most trouble to individual groups are shown in Appendix 3. Cows' milk and food colouring came top of the list but the letters disclosed that many innocent seeming foods had come under suspicion. These individual foods and the symptoms they are believed to have caused are described throughout the book.

The letters also revealed that a food which causes breathing difficulties in one person may not cause it in another. However the same food may cause a different complaint, say a skin rash, in a third person. There seems no rule as to which food causes any particular allergy. Although cows' milk may cause more trouble than other foods, just because it is found to be the cause of one person's problem does not mean that cutting it out will automatically help someone else suffering from the same complaint. You may be discarding a valuable food unnecessarily. You must discover for yourself whether cows' milk is the cause of your complaint.

The letters came from ordinary men and women. Either they or their children were the sufferers. Some had made their discoveries with the help of a doctor, either their GP or one at a NHS hospital, some privately at allergy clinics and some by just observing their reactions and working out the solution for themselves. Others were helped by self-help organisations dealing with their particular complaint.

The fear of being labelled a hypochondriac or food crank was repeatedly voiced. Many people said how pleased they were that the subject had been brought out into the open and allowed them to feel that they were not the only ones thinking along these lines. The letters and examples quoted throughout this book are representative of people suffering from food allergy; they are not representative of the population as a whole.

Ignorance about food allergy is rife. A letter from the membership secretary of a local branch of the Asthma Society in 1983 sums it up: 'Not having heard of particular foods being associated with asthma, I shall be most interested in the book you are writing. At our next open meeting I shall read out your letter as I am sure our members and friends will be interested in your discovery.' This letter shows the need for a much wider awareness of the connection between food and allergies – an awareness by both the medical profession and the public at large.

## My discovery

My son suffers from asthma and used to get eczema. One winter evening when he was five he was playing with a friend in our sitting room, absorbed in what he was doing but wheezing loudly. His friend's mother had just arrived and on seeing me walk into the room carrying a bottle of Heinz tomato ketchup (I was in the middle of preparing supper) announced 'You realise you are poisoning your child giving him that stuff.' I was horrified and furious. How dare someone say I was harming my own son. Then when he asked for a drink of milk, her look spoke volumes. 'You don't give him milk, do you? You know asthmatics should not drink milk.'

I decided to test her views. I stopped my son drinking milk and eating dairy products for two weeks. He was still very wheezy. The lady was wrong: he was not allergic to either milk or tomato ketchup (not the Heinz brand anyway). But she made me think about what he had been eating and why he had been so wheezy for many days, needing medicines regularly, sometimes three or four times a day.

My husband hit upon it. We thought back to when this present bout had started and what he had been eating and drinking. Cola drink was the answer. We stopped giving him it. He immediately started to improve and became clear for some weeks. Then suddenly he started to wheeze again. Why? We thought again and I realised I had started to give him a hot chocolate drink when he returned from school. I stopped the chocolate drink. The wheezing stopped. We then decided to chart what he ate and how he was. Whenever he had some chocolate or cola drink, he would wheeze for some three to four days after, usually needing medicine. The attack would reach a peak after about 24 hours and then take another two or three days to subside. There could be no doubt. These foods were making him ill.

Conclusive proof of the cola drink as a cause of his asthma came completely by mistake. On holiday, my son had been clear of any symptoms for over two weeks. We were staying overnight with some American friends and that late afternoon were offered some drinks. 'Would you like a lemon soda?' my friend asked and I gratefully accepted. It did not taste like lemon but I took a few sips and left the rest. My son then enquired what it was and drank it. Four hours later he started to wheeze. What was the cause? We racked our brains. Nothing he had eaten could have triggered off the attack. 'What about that drink?' asked my husband, having returned from soothing our son at about three in the morning. We rummaged through the rubbish bin and found no lemon soda can but a cola can. The following morning we asked our friend what the drink had been and she confirmed that it was cola.

Since then we have discovered he is allergic to other foods or rather additives contained within them. A fresh home-made hamburger is okay, a frozen one is not (if it contains the flavour enhancer monosodium glutamate (621) which many do). Natural ice creams can be easily eaten, ice creams with added colour make him wheeze. The list grew. Whenever tartrazine (a yellow food colouring coded E102) or monosodium glutamate appeared in the ingredients, he would have an attack.

## Can it be true?

It may be difficult to believe that a food or drink which does not cause a stomach upset can sometimes cause severe symptoms in your head, nose, chest or skin. Sceptics doubt there is anything in it; they say food is not the cause of allergic symptoms. But 30 years ago, few people agreed that cigarettes were a danger to health. Now cigarettes are banned from advertising on television and have a health warning on every packet and press advertisement.

Only a few clinical studies have been undertaken which prove that foods cause allergies. There is probably a good reason for this. As one doctor told me 'We might have a strong suspicion that a food is causing an allergy in a patient but to prove conclusively that an allergy exists you have to give a patient repeated doses of the suspected food to make sure that it really is making him ill. And who wants to become repeatedly ill for the sake of science and to prove a point?' Dr Theron Randolph, an American doctor and allergy specialist says that in his experience, food allergy is one of the greatest health problems in the USA. He has treated 20,000 patients for food allergies and related problems and has dealt with virtually every kind of chronic illness on an allergic basis.[1]

## Consult your doctor

If you or one of your family is ill, you seek help from your doctor: and quite rightly so. A doctor takes the emergency out of a situation and tries to sort out what the problem is. He will probably prescribe drugs to cure or at least calm the complaint.

But what happens if the complaint persists; or comes back regularly. And your doctor cannot find a cure to stop the symptoms returning or an adequate reason as to why they should occur in the first place. Then begins the constant trek to the surgery and probably to your local hospital. If one drug does not seem to be effective, stronger drugs may be prescribed. The symptoms may be relieved but the cause still remains.

At this stage you should think seriously about the cause. Could it be an allergy? And if so, to what? Dr Richard Mackarness has tentatively estimated that 30 per cent of people attending GPs have symptoms traceable exclusively to food and chemical allergy; 30 per cent have symptoms partially traceable to this cause, and the remaining 40 per cent have symptoms which are unrelated to allergy.[2]

Unfortunately there are some doctors who do not believe food can cause allergies and others who may not have enough knowledge to help you. Here are some typical examples:

Helen, a doctor's daughter herself, found her doctor unhelpful. 'My GP just labelled me as a neurotic.' Her son aged three suffers from asthma. He is allergic to tartrazine (E102), a yellow food colouring, which she says she finally proved when her son had an attack six hours after eating jelly containing the dye. Her question, and one repeated by many, is 'Why don't hospitals suggest food as a cause?'

Caroline echoes Helen's point and also found tartrazine to be the offending ingredient. Her son is six years old and has suffered from both asthma and eczema. 'He was never without a boil or abcess somewhere on his body – he was so painfully thin and tired the whole family were affected as we were up every single night with him. The medical treatment he was having was no help. He was in and out of hospital where they made him well but not for long.'

Caroline read a magazine article about the yellow colouring tartrazine which described all the symptoms her son had. It also listed many foods containing it. 'James drank a lot of Robinsons orange drink and so I wrote to Colmans, the manufacturers, to see if it contained E102 (the code number by which tartrazine is usually described). They very kindly sent me a list of all their foods with E102 added – which included their orange drink. We have watched James' diet very closely since and there is a marked change in his health: he now has a good attendance at school and is able to concentrate, although I would say that he is still not quite right. One thing I cannot understand (and I will ask the doctor at the hospital on James' next visit) is since they have known about the effects of tartrazine on sensitive folk for some while – why were we not asked to test this out?' Colman's has subsequently removed tartrazine (E102) from Robinson's Whole Orange Drink and now uses two other artificial colours, sunset yellow (E110) and quinoline yellow (E104).

Gizella's parents were told off by their doctor for being difficult and insinuations were made that they were causing a psychological problem. Gizella is a teenager who often suffered from migraine attacks which made her look 30. She was told to relax and take headache tablets. She has since discovered she is allergic to some additives found in many foods: monosodium glutamate (621), sodium nitrate (E251) and other preservatives. She also cannot eat tomatoes or citrus fruit like oranges and grapefruit.

## Help yourself

If your doctor thinks you, or your child, has an allergy, he may refer you to an allergy clinic, either through the National Health Service or privately. You will need a letter from your doctor to consult a hospital specialist. At the clinic, you, or your child, may be given tests (see p. 87) and if the patient is thought to be allergic to foods, may be put on some sort of food elimination diet. More drugs may be prescribed.

A small number of doctors, who specialise in allergies caused by food and chemicals, are called clinical ecologists. Although thin on the ground and usually private which means paying sometimes high fees, you can obtain the name of one who practises nearest to you by sending a stamped self-addressed envelope to Action Against Allergy or contacting the National Society for Research into Allergy. The British Society for Allergy and Environmental Medicine supplies a list of doctors specialising in allergy but not necessarily food allergy. The addresses of these organisations are given in Appendix 1.

But unfortunately some doctors, even specialists, may not believe food causes allergies. If your doctor shrugs his shoulders sceptically or pats you kindly on the head, do not accept his attitude. You have nothing to lose by testing out your theories yourself, provided you go about it sensibly.

Janet did not accept the advice of her doctor and health visitor that her son was frustrated and would grow out of it. Since birth he had been unsettled. He cried constantly, was never still and slept little. 'Four years later still waiting for an improvement I happened to speak to a playgroup leader who knew of a girl who was hyperactive and on a special diet eliminating colourings, flavourings and preservatives. I tried this diet with amazing results. The crying stopped and he calmed down almost immediately. He became a pal whereas before we had had constant battles.'

Debbie complained that she had found it hard to get the hospital doctors' co-operation when she wanted to try her two and a half year old son on a diet to help rid him of his bad eczema. Eventually after much nagging, they referred her to a dietician who proved most helpful. She eliminated dairy produce, squash, tap water and cocoa and says, a year later, he is 80 per cent better.

Many people have found out the cause of their allergy for themselves. You can too. Seek advice and guidance from your doctor or local hospital, but do not be afraid to search out the answer for yourself. You are in control of your own, or your child's body, every day. You can observe symptoms and their changes much more closely than any medical team and, except in the case of a very acute attack, you can deal with them as effectively.

Ted is a good example of someone discovering the cause of his headaches by thinking about what he ate: 'For many years I suffered from headaches, diagnosed as migraine, but could not believe that psychological reasons were the cause. Eventually I decided to treat the complaint by controlling my diet. This followed a period when a headache was suffered each Wednesday afternoon. On Wednesdays I visited the same restaurant and had the roast lunch. At first I tried boiled potatoes in place of roast ones – but no change. Then I varied the vegetables, sauce etc., and eventually found the cause was the Yorkshire pudding which was served with regular monotony with every roast.'

Ted is not sure what it is in the Yorkshire pudding which triggered off his migraine but he has learned to leave it on his plate. He also gets headaches from tinned chocolate pudding, batter from fish and chips and artificial cream. He has not pinpointed what it is in these foods which causes his migraine but he does not eat them and feels a lot better.

## Is the medicine necessary?

Do you need to take so much medicine? Or are you just calming the effects of something you can actually prevent. Many people, both medical and lay, feel the Western world reaches too readily for a bottle of medicine to find the solution.

In the case of Sue's son he would have been spared many doses of penicillin and much discomfort if milk had been diagnosed, or at least suspected earlier, of causing his asthma. She writes: 'When my second son was ten days old, he developed what my health visitor diagnosed as the snuffles. His snuffles then became bronchitis which had the added complication of an ear infection. A course of penicillin was prescribed and his condition improved. Within about two weeks the symptoms returned and this pattern continued until he was about nine months old.

'My own doctor was convinced it was something he would grow out of but after about ten courses of penicillin we insisted on him being referred to the local hospital. The doctor diagnosed asthma and gave him the necessary medicine. After a month we returned as he was no better and saw another doctor who thought that the asthma was caused by an allergy. As he was bottle fed she thought that the allergy must be caused by milk. Milk was then taken from his diet completely and he was like a different child. Providing he has no milk at all in his diet, he is completely free of asthma and all the side effects.'

Professor Lino Businco of the University of Rome has stated[3] that asthma can be caused by a 'flu virus which releases histamine in the lungs. He said that prescribing antibiotics was of no use whatsoever and that if necessary an anti-asthma drug should be taken.

A lady from Wales objected to her hospital's advice to use more drugs on her asthmatic son and like Sue found an alternative solution by cutting out cows' milk. She writes: 'I have two children, a girl aged nine and a boy Lloyd aged seven, both asthma sufferers. This winter has proved a particularly bad one for Lloyd and I forever seemed to be calling out doctors to see him but of course as he was already on medicine they said they could do nothing more for him. The hospital prescribed steroid treatment for him but I was against this for one so young. I was told however that if he was not better by next check-up, then there would be no alternative but to put him on steroid treatment.

'Three weeks ago I was so desperate (Lloyd was having attacks practically every hour throughout the night), I went to a herbalist. He told me to stop giving him milk or anything containing milk or dairy products immediately. I tried this together with some herbal tablets he recommended and the difference in Lloyd in just three weeks is really amazing. His attacks are down to just one on most nights and he looks so well. I find it so hard to believe that none of the dozens of doctors we have seen with Lloyd and his sister have ever been able to suggest this before.'

Finally Janette, and even more so her small son, would have been spared much trouble and the use of sedatives if the cause of his disturbed nights had been detected earlier. She writes: 'My elder son aged three was a sort of coiled spring, forever rushing about, unable to be still for any length of time. From Christmas 1981, the only undisturbed nights we had were when he was drugged; it was not at all unusual for him to get up 12 to 14 times a night, and he became used to any sedative within a couple of days.

'We assumed that it was some sort of belated jealous reaction to the new baby born in August 1981. We tried all combinations of advice and finally in desperation and a lot of scepticism, I cut out all forms of preservatives, colourings and additives. My health visitor said that it would take four days for the existing 'poisons' to be eliminated and on the fourth night he slept right through. The change was dramatic. He also has a tendency to 'chestiness', patchy eczema and has an allergy to something we have yet to discover: these have not altered but compared to the wild-eyed maniac I used to have, they are minor irritations.'

If you feel you have found the cause of your own, or your child's allergy, and get better, you may consider reducing the medicine taken and eventually stopping it if you, or your child, stay well. Consult your doctor first and tell him what you intend to do as with some drugs it can be dangerous to stop the dose suddenly. If you get worse again, you will probably want to take a drug to relieve the symptoms. But at least give it a try.

## Homoeopathy

While considering what alternatives there are to prescribed drugs, you may wish to visit a doctor who practises homoeopathy. Although qualified in conventional medicine, their approach is often quite different from a GP's. Some homoeopaths are not qualified doctors. A first consultation may last from half an hour to an hour and you will be asked many questions not only about your condition but how you feel generally, your moods, in fact 'what makes you tick'. One patient who consulted a homoeopath came away saying 'I felt my soul was being searched'.

The basis of homoeopathy is that the patient is treated and not just the disease. Questions may concern your past health and family circumstances, the pattern of health in your family and your present condition. There are also questions about your personality. Do you prefer hot or cold weather, the sea or the mountains? Are you musical or artistic, quick-tempered or sulky? What are your hopes, fears and aspirations? At the end of the consultation, the homoeopath has drawn up a mental picture of the patient and may then recommend a remedy. The remedy is made from one of a number of natural substances which is taken in the form of a pill, tablet, powder or lotion. The size and frequency of the dose varies according to each patient.

I took my son to a homoeopathic doctor who prescribed him what looked like tiny round white sugar pills which had been impregnated with such a remedy. He was told to take one every two hours whenever he had an asthmatic attack. I was very sceptical that these would work but tried them out. They did work and for two years my son took one of his 'little white pills' whenever he had an attack. Often one homoeopathic pill was sufficient but if necessary another was taken two hours later. Subsequently we found these homoeopathic pills less effective but then on such occasions when he had a severe attack nor was the prescribed conventional medicine fully effective.

Many people claim they have been helped by taking homoeopathic medicine; others have found it of no use. Homoeopathic treatment can be obtained within the National Health Service but only to a limited extent. Most doctors practise privately. The British Homoeopathic Association publishes a list of doctors, both NHS and private, practising homoeopathy throughout the UK (see Appendix 1 for address).

## Your discovery

There are many ways you can go about trying to discover if food is, or is not, causing your or your child's allergy. But if you want to make a start, here and now, I suggest you keep a diary listing everything you eat, drink and how you feel. By noting down all these details every day and by using your observation and commonsense, you may discover, with the help of this book, if there is any link between what you eat and how you feel. You will discover what foods you can eat as well as any you cannot. The diary will show the good periods as well as the bad. It may seem an endless and awesome task but it is not. It takes only five minutes every evening (or any other time of the day) to keep a diary and certainly in my son's case it has proved invaluable.

The necessity of keeping a diary is that it is almost impossible to recall exactly how you felt or what you ate even a few days ago, let alone weeks ago. Try to remember exactly what you ate during the past three days. I am sure you cannot. But if you can do that, try to remember what you ate for supper three Mondays ago. Unless it was your birthday or a special occasion, I bet you will find this impossible. It is not difficult to chart your, or your child's, health and what has been eaten. This is explained in Chapter 3. It is also not difficult to read the ingredients on packaging to find out what the food contains, even if it takes more time. Keep and date the labels, if necessary, to refer to, see Chapter 4.

If you suspect a food, eliminate it. But do not cut out too many foods at once. It may be unnecessary and could be harmful if not adequately replaced with other equally nutritious food. Guidelines on how to go about this are given in Chapter 3. One man's meat is another man's poison. This is the message I aim to get across in this book. Your poison may not be as widespread as you think and may be avoidable. The important thing to remember is that a particular food which may cause such distress to one person can be totally beneficial to another.

## Is it in the family?

If there is someone in your family suffering from an allergy, it should make you aware that your, or your child's, condition could also be one. But neither the symptoms nor the cause of them need be the same. Just because Dad has hayfever caused by grass pollen, this does not mean that son's asthma is caused by the same irritant; it could be another pollen or it could be a food. Do not rely on allergies or the same allergy running in families. Although I received many letters saying that more than one member of the family suffered from the same or different symptoms, there were other letters saying no-one else in the family seemed to be afflicted.

Margaret has suffered from allergies for most of her life but her daughters fortunately do not: 'As a baby, I suffered from eczema. This grew worse and it was not until my early twenties when I had allergy tests that it was discovered I was allergic, amongst other things, to cows' milk. I stopped drinking all milk and had an immediate improvement although I am still affected by cat and dog hair, dust, pollen and wool. In my early forties, I seemed to get worse, suffering from a blotchy rash to arms, face, neck and also parts of my body. The irritation was intense and I had further allergy tests only to be told that I had now developed a further allergy to sugar and monosodium glutamate (621). I have two daughters who seem to have escaped this problem.'

Bernard on the other hand has found that he and his two children get wheezy as a result of eating wheat and sugar in different combinations. Elizabeth discovered that she and her children are allergic to eggs; all suffer from a form of eczema when this 'culprit' food is eaten.

## Finding the culprit

Your sense of achievement, as well as relief, when you discover a food 'culprit' will be great. As was Georgina's when she helped her son. She writes: 'Barry is seven years old, sturdy and top of his class at school but his allergies are now controlled. It was a different picture before this was achieved. His food and drug allergy first presented itself on being given penicillin – severe ulceration of his mouth. The drug was withdrawn and the condition resolved. As a toddler he was constantly suffering from urticaria (nettlerash) and periods when his whole personality changed, becoming unco-ordinated, falling over, crying, irritable and generally unwell.

'My GP was not too helpful, so having a family history of migraine and hayfever, I decided to read up on all the information available re food allergies and withdrew all suspect foods from the diet, gradually reintroducing all suspect food, noting very interesting results. The old symptoms returned when any of the following were taken: white flour, chocolate (hard on a child this), monosodium glutamate, artificial colourings, additives, preservatives, citric acid (Vitamin C), acetic acid. Any carbonated drink, especially cola. Ice cream and treacle cause headaches, milk causes a runny nose if taken in excess. Having found Barry's tolerance level of these foods, the occasional treat is permissible.

'I was delighted that I was able to control the problems myself and this has compensated for the extra time planning menus, reading labels and lengthy explanations to hosts when refusing food and drink; a small price to pay for the health of one's child.'

## Not everyone's answer

Allergic symptoms may be caused by irritants other than food. Pollen, mould spores, dust and housedust mites; environmental pollution such as gas and petrol fumes; fabrics both natural and man-made; and cosmetics and washing aids may well affect you adversely (see p. 82 for more details). Emotional upsets may also encourage allergies to appear.

Food, either eating or not eating it, is not the miracle cure for all medical problems. It is important to establish that your symptoms are not caused by other illnesses and it is therefore necessary to consult your doctor, especially if you get symptoms you have not had before. But if your doctor cannot cure you and you suspect food may be the answer, test it out. If you are successful in pinpointing a food or foods, show the evidence to your doctor. It may convert him into believing what may be for him a new idea; and this may help many future patients.

There is nothing to be lost and everything to be gained by applying the advice in this book to discovering whether you, or your child, may be allergic to a food. Please give it a try.

### Notes

1 *An Alternative Approach to Allergies*, Theron G. Randolph MD and Ralph W. Moss PhD, Bantam Books, 1980. Published in the UK by Thorsons.
2 *Not All in the Mind*, Dr Richard Mackarness, Pan Books, 1976, p.37.
3 Action Against Allergy Public Symposium, London, June 1984.

# 2

# What is an allergy?

A food allergy is the appearance of any unpleasant symptoms as a result of something you eat or drink. The most common complaints are detailed in this chapter.

Some doctors argue that when a food causes you to suffer a bad reaction, for example migraine (headache) or stomach upset, you may not be allergic to that food but *intolerant* of it or *hypersensitive* to it. These differences may help medical researchers and chemists try to discover the reason why certain people react and others do not, but until a safe way is found of preventing a bad reaction, whether you are allergic, intolerant or hypersensitive to a food or drink, makes no difference to the sufferer. If you avoid that food, you do not get that reaction: the medical distinction does not help. Throughout this book all these conditions are described as allergies. Some doctors may suggest that you have a psychological aversion to a food. I would ignore this suggestion. If you feel better after not eating a certain food, avoid that food.

Certain conditions, when food has to be restricted or forbidden, are not allergies. These include heart disease and high blood pressure where often a low fat or low salt diet is recommended by doctors. Another is diabetes when a low intake of sugar is essential and a high fibre diet recommended.[1] People who are diagnosed as suffering from coeliac disease (irritation of the small intestine) are told to avoid gluten found in wheat and other cereals and recent research has shown that the elimination of milk and dairy products can help sufferers of ulcerative colitis (a condition which causes severe stomach pains).

The name of an allergy may vary although the symptoms are the same: doctors may give a medical title to symptoms which can be explained more simply. For example, what one person may describe as a headache, another might describe as migraine. Someone might be described as wheezy, another as asthmatic. Another suffering from eczema may describe it as a horrible rash. The names are different but the discomfort to the sufferer is the same.

The following allergies are described so that those connected with breathing come together, as do skin complaints, headaches and so on. Examples from the letters I received are also quoted. A table of some of the major foods causing these conditions is printed in Appendix 3. You may just want to read about the symptoms you, or a member of your family, suffer from and skip the rest of this chapter.

## Allergies which may be caused by food

**Breathing or respiratory conditions**
Common cold symptoms
Runny or blocked nose (rhinitis, catarrh)
Sore eyes (conjunctivitis)
Sneezing
Thick feeling in head
Hayfever – any or all of the above symptoms
Wheezing (asthma)

**Skin conditions**
Eczema
Rashes (hives, nettlerash, urticaria)
Swelling of face or body
Mouth ulcers

**Headaches**
Migraine

**Hyperactivity in children**
Unusual, unruly behaviour

**Bedwetting and lack of bladder control**

**Stomach upsets**
Indigestion
Cramps
Feeling sick (nausea)
Being sick (vomiting)
Diarrhoea

**Depression and nightmares in adults**

**Aches, pains and arthritis**

**Fits and convulsions**

## The common cold

What is the 'common cold'? What are the symptoms? Runny or blocked up nose, sore eyes, sneezing, sore throat, a thick feeling in the head. How often do you hear people describe any of these symptoms and moan 'I have had this cold for ages and can't seem to shrug it off'. Your doctor may give it a fancy title:

- catarrh – a blocked nose
- rhinitis – a runny nose
- conjunctivitis – sore, inflamed eyes
- hayfever – runny nose, streaming eyes, sneezing, inflamed throat

However most people will associate these symptoms with that well known and often experienced British complaint – the common cold. Is it caused by a virus? Is it caused by something you are breathing like grass pollen or air pollution? Or is it being caused by something you eat or drink? Consult your doctor and see what he says. Hayfever caused by pollen can be alleviated by medicines and infections may need to be treated with drugs. But I feel that people too readily rely on drugs and should allow their own bodies to cope with minor ailments. If you take a medicine for five days, how can you be sure it was the medicine which cured you: you may have got better anyway. This idea may be considered controversial but is worth a thought. If you do not get better, you can always reconsider at any time and seek medical aid.

## Runny or blocked nose

If you are suffering from a perpetual cold or one which seems to come back frequently, you may need to look to food or some other irritant for the cause.

John found that dairy produce caused his chronic allergic rhinitis (a continuously runny nose). He says that other foods which aggravate the condition are curry and alcohol and reports that avoiding these foods 'minimises a permanent, unpleasant and never-ending affliction'. Judith said that full-cream cows' milk, but not skimmed milk, produces heavy catarrh (a blocked nose) within 24 hours.

Rosemary, aged 46, discovered that chicken, beef, eggs and dairy produce caused her 'cold'. 'I have had cold type symptoms, wheeziness and itchy eyes for years and years and put up with them. Since I have kept off various foods, I have been very much better and off all the tablets and sprays that I was having.' Jill found that white sugar and sugar substitutes made her sneeze violently and gave her a runny nose. And Gladys found chocolate gives her 'a terrible catarrh'. The daughter of a lady from Lincolnshire found that 'alcohol of any kind makes her sneeze, her eyes run, with a generally bunged up feeling'; Pat on the other hand found eggs make her feel fluey: 'The only way I can describe this reaction. Sometimes a dull headache, aching joints'.

## Hayfever

This complaint is usually associated with an allergy to grass pollen but can be caused by many other plants and trees (see p. 85). It can also be caused by food.

Joan's husband used to sneeze and have a runny nose every ten days or so for one whole day and had to take tablets for it. Two years ago they discovered he is allergic to onions and by avoiding them rarely gets it now. He can eat garlic and dried onions but when he tried frozen onions recently he had the usual symptoms for over an hour. The fact that you get a runny nose and eyes while cutting fresh onions is well-known.

Sarah's daughter, aged five, developed very bad hayfever except that it continued after the grass pollen season had ended. Sarah writes of her daughter: 'She had red, swollen, itchy eyes, runny nose always congested, sneezing. Nose drops, eye drops, preventative nose spray, anti-histamine medicine did nothing except threaten to make her into a mini-hypochondriac: "Is it time for my drops/spray/medicine yet, Mummy?" Doctors just advised putting up with it and could do no more. She was desperately uncomfortable and not sleeping at nights.

'I took out of her diet all things containing artificial colouring, flavouring, preservatives, stabilisers etc., and also all refined foods such as white sugar, white flour and white breakfast cereals. Within a week, she did not need any of her treatments and last summer during the hayfever season we did not have to visit the doctor at all. We find now that if she eats or drinks what we call 'rubbish' it affects her during the night after – she wakes up with a totally blocked up nose and then the other symptoms follow and she feels a general malaise; it usually takes about 48 hours to get her back to normal.'

Dorothy's 'cold' was cured by her doctor but not with medicine: 'About three years ago, I suffered from an allergy for about ten months. The effect was like a continuous bout of hayfever, watery eyes and nose and a feeling of being unable to breathe properly. My doctor, who also himself suffered from a similar allergy, advised me to go on a 'no cereal diet'. This meant having nothing made with flour and the only cereal allowed was sago. What could I eat in place of bread? My doctor advised potatoes in all forms and even gave me a recipe for pastry using potato flour. At that time I ate a lot of potato crisps. Well, the result was after a few weeks on this diet, I was cured of my allergy and am now back to an almost normal diet except I still do not eat any breakfast cereals.'

## Asthma

This condition occurs when the muscles around the air passages in the lungs contract and the lining of the air passages swells. This hinders the flow of air into and out of the lungs. Extra mucus may also be produced. Wheezing (the noise made by air being forced through the narrowed space) usually occurs when breathing out but may also happen when breathing in. Wheezing may provoke coughing and coughing may aggravate the sensitivity of the lungs which in turn causes more wheezing. Asthma can be accompanied by headaches, vomiting and even a fever. There are two million asthma sufferers in Britain.

Asthma can be caused by many irritants: pollen, mould spores, house dust mites, air pollution, for example; but food and drink must be taken into account. Yellow and orange food colouring used in many foods including squash and sweets, milk and dairy produce, sugar and wheat seem common offenders although almost any food may be the culprit.

Helen found that many milk-based products caused her to suffer asthma; they produced a very bad tightening of the chest. Two people wrote to say that yeast brought on an attack.

Chloe aged four was able to spend a very pleasant winter last year with no asthma attacks when her mother stopped her drinking or eating anything with orange colouring in it. Her mother wrote: 'The difference is amazing compared to the previous winter when she could not walk, eat, play etc. Nothing seemed to help her.' Chloe still takes some medicine but finds she needs it less and less.

Mavis developed asthma at the age of 19. It gradually increased in severity until her forties when it was very bad indeed: 'I had to take steroid drug courses and tried numerous inhalers and other tablets. Also had bronchitis[2] many times, very rarely sleeping through the night when it was usually at its worst. The steroid drugs also caused me to put on a lot of weight. I weighed $12\frac{1}{2}$ stone and I am 5 ft 4 in tall. I was quite desperate by the time I was 52. My doctor said I must try very hard to lose weight. I really made a great effort and cut out bread, flour products, potatoes and sugar. In a couple of days a miracle happened. My asthma abruptly stopped altogether. Afer 33 years it stopped and I have not had another attack in the last five years. I lost three and a half stone and feel at least 15 years younger – no bronchitis either in the last five years or even a cold. I just feel marvellous. I can only surmise that I am allergic to wheat products though I have not proved this. I take no medicine at all and sleep well.'

Egg gave Carol's son asthma and a streaming nose within ten minutes; and a dab of egg white on his skin produced a welt within a couple of minutes. He can tolerate eggs cooked with other foods but never eats whole egg on its own. Peanuts also produce a violent reaction; asthma, nettlerash and vomiting. Even a trace of peanuts in a food gives him indigestion and itches. Milk products have also caused problems in the past but he can now eat them in small doses. He is aged nine. Carol went on to mention that food colouring, additives and preservatives made little or no difference which once again goes to show that one man's meat is another man's poison.

Both children and adults suffer from asthma but Maura was stunned when as she puts it: 'I found myself reduced from a human dynamo to a listless snuffler at the age of 32. I had no childhood asthma, was not a smoker, drinker or overweight.' She improved with standard treatment but still found life looking after her husband and five year old son together with a full time job a considerable strain. She persuaded a locum (a stand-in for her local doctor) to put her forward for full allergy testing in the local hospital. 'Rudimentary skin testing revealed only a slight reaction to milk and fish. I was very disappointed but was so desperately worried as to whether I could continue working that I decided never to eat either again or any of their derivatives. Within a week I felt slightly better and after three weeks I knew that the improvement was no illusion. Now although still under the same medical treatment, my condition has markedly improved.'

## Eczema

An irritating, disfiguring and often painful skin condition which affects millions of men, women and children, eczema derives its name from the Greek verb *ekzema* which means to boil. There are at least fourteen different types of eczema. Sufferers tend to have an itchy skin and develop patches of red rash which sometimes become raw or weeping. In extreme cases, the rash can cover most of the body and may be accompanied by small blisters which burst when the skin is scratched to relieve itching. Eczema is neither infectious nor contagious.[3]

Based on the results of a national follow-up of all five-year-olds born in Great Britain during 5–11 April 1970, a report by the Department of Child Health in Bristol showed that over 12 per cent of the children had suffered from eczema. For the majority the condition had appeared before they were four years old and more than half had stopped having symptoms by the time they were five.

The study seems to indicate that breast-feeding does not protect children against eczema: 13·2 per cent of babies who were breast-fed during their first week of life developed eczema later compared with 10·9 per cent who were bottle-fed. In general the longer the child was breast-fed, the more likely he or she was to have eczema. However there was a significantly higher risk amongst those children who were both breast-fed and given some form of supplementary feed.

Whether children are protected against having eczema by being breast-fed is a much researched subject which as yet seems undecided. The results of the Bristol study seem to contradict most doctors' belief that breast-feeding is better for such conditions (and is healthier in general). If a baby is highly susceptible to allergy, its mother should also take care of her diet so that no food likely to cause trouble can be passed through her own milk to her baby.

Eczema can be caused by almost any food or drink although milk, wheat, eggs, food colouring and some fruits seem to be the worst offenders.

Hazel's son suffered from eczema which covered a sizeable part of his body when it was at its worst. A friend who was a nurse suggested that cows' milk might be the cause. She fed her son goats' milk instead and the results, she says, were most impressive.

Pauline, on the other hand, found that milk was not the cause of her son's eczema. He had suffered from eczema since the age of nine months and Pauline's doctor suggested that milk might be the cause of his allergy, especially as it had started just after she had finished breast-feeding. She cut out milk but it made no difference at all. 'I then started treating him with hydrocortisone ointments and oily bath additives prescribed by the doctor. But I was not very happy doing that because I wanted to find the cause. I systematically cut out various foods until I discovered which suited him and which did not. I now try and avoid tomatoes, rhubarb, strawberries, beetroot and red food colouring. These all trigger an attack of eczema.'

Eve, now aged 60, discovered that eggs, white flour, tomatoes and shellfish caused her to suffer eczema on her face and neck from the age of 15. She says: 'I took anti-histamine tablets for a few years but gave them up because they made me very drowsy. I now try to avoid the foods to which I am allergic.'

Citrus fruit such as oranges and grapefruit can be another culprit for some people. Louise has suffered from both asthma and eczema since she was 18 months old. She is now 12 and has received all kinds of drugs and treatments for both. Her mother discovered that satsumas and oranges made her extremely sore. It was not any contact on the skin that was the problem. It was the eating of the oranges that made her skin itch and erupt. Her mother writes: 'We cut out all citrus fruit and have noticed quite a difference. Very few restless nights, scratching approximately four or five times in a year compared with almost daily. The doctor at the hospital said it was just coincidence but we tried at various intervals, sometimes two weeks, sometimes three months, and every time she had an orange she was very sore the following day; enough evidence for us to believe what we saw.'

It need not be oranges themselves which cause this distressing complaint. It may be the orange colouring used in many manufactured foods to give them such a vivid colour.

Michael was born with infantile eczema but this disappeared after his first year. It then reappeared in his second/third years and persisted despite frequent treatments by his GP. When he was five, his mother read a report from America about the bad effects of colouring used in foods and orange drinks. She tells: 'Michael has always drunk a lot of orange squash. The rather vivid colour had worried me for a little time and after reading the American report, we switched him to pure orange juice. The eczema of years disappeared within days never to return – except that, when he was about nine, he was given a glass or two of the discontinued squash, by mischance, and promptly came out in the old eczema. We quickly stopped the squash and he promptly recovered and has not suffered again.'

About eight years ago, Zania developed a form of eczema on her scalp which made most of her hair fall out. Different doctors and specialists tried various creams and lotions without success so eventually she went to see a trichologist (an unqualified hair 'doctor'). He advised her to stop drinking coffee (she drank about four cups a day) but said tea was okay. Within a few weeks the eczema had cleared up and her hair started to grow again. She says: 'To prove the point, about three years ago I went on holiday and could not get tea to drink, only coffee and chocolate. I chose coffee and the eczema started within two days. I immediately changed to chocolate and my scalp cleared up. Needless to say, I do not drink coffee any more.'

Dr David Atherton, a children's skin specialist, writes in a booklet prepared for the National Eczema Society[4]: 'We do now have fairly strong evidence that foods are a major cause of eczema.

In fact it has been shown in careful studies that as many as two out of every three children with eczema will benefit from a simple manipulation of the diet . . . Although almost any food appears able to provoke eczema, two stand out from the crowd; they are eggs and milk. In my hospital, we often ask children who are avoiding egg and milk to avoid chicken at the same time.' Dr Atherton goes on to say: 'Reactions to artificial colours and preservatives in foods appear so common that it may be a good idea to include these in the elimination, even if one has no other reason to suspect them. After egg and milk, they seem to be the next most important dietary factors in eczema.'

## Rashes

This section includes rashes which do not come under the heading of eczema. My survey shows that they can be caused by many foods or additives as well as by cosmetics, household goods, too much sun or heat and drugs. Here are a few examples of rashes caused by different foods:

Phyllis's youngest son, aged eight months, had a reaction within ten minutes of eating an egg yolk. The skin surrounding his mouth became bright red followed by a rash (like a nettlerash). After a bout of vomiting, his whole body suffered the same reaction. This lasted for about three hours.

Peggy found that green vegetables caused an irritation around her eyelashes which later spread all over her body. It seems to her that the crunchy spine and stalk of a lettuce causes more harm than the other parts of the leaf.

Food colouring also appears to cause trouble in some people. Connie developed a severe rash soon after she married. It was an angry pink which covered her from head to toe and included swelling of her ankles and lips. After unsuccessful treatment from her doctor she was referred to a hospital consultant and put on a diet for six weeks, sampling different foods. Tartrazine (E102), a yellow colouring in many foods, was the cause of the rash.

Clinical studies have shown that a variety of food additives can cause urticaria.[5] Urticaria is the medical name for slightly raised, smooth, flat-topped weals which appear on the skin. They may be redder or paler than the surrounding skin but often resemble mosquito bites.

Joan used to get 'chocolate spots': they were disfiguring red raised blotches with a white centre which would last for days. She says: 'I used to eat lots of chocolate. One day a patient I was X-raying recognised them and thankfully said spontaneously "chocolate spots". I have never had a chocolate since and no more spots.'

Muriel discovered that gluten found in wheat and other cereals (see p. 75) brought her out in a severe skin irritation with slight red marks, especially on her arms.

## Face and body swelling

I received several letters saying these conditions were caused by a food or foods. Barbara writes: 'Periodically my mouth and cheeks would swell. Within about half an hour I became a very grotesque sight. Also on several occasions my tongue would swell almost to the feeling of it going to choke me. I had to go immediately to the doctor who gave me an injection.' Barbara tried eliminating many foods without success. It was eventually suggested by a friend that celery might be the cause. Barbara says: 'Although I have not had any tests I have not eaten any celery since, which is now about four years ago and had no allergy.'

Bridget claims it is the combination of vanilla and orange which makes her face swell like a football and the rest of her body to a lesser extent. 'The effect of the combination is that I begin to itch (usually starting in the corner of the eyes) and then "heat bumps" appear and spread to join up. My face swells up like a football. My nose disappears as the swelling is so great and very often there are two or three folds of flesh on my cheeks. During a bad attack I have physically to hold my eyes open to see. The swelling is not so evident over the rest of my body although the "heat bumps" spread everywhere.'

Sylvia says that over the last three to four years she has become allergic to green food colouring. 'It was not too difficult to pinpoint the cause. The day after eating some green jelly, my eyes suddenly became like a frog's, discoloured and lined. It made me look about 90 and was a very depressing experience. Since then, each time I have eaten anything containing green food colouring, such as manufactured mint sauce or tinned peas, my eyes have reacted in the same way.'

To emphasise the point that a food which affects one person may not affect another, Fred wrote about his youngest son, a twin. 'In summer he would often swell around the eyes and a jelly would form over them. He would eventually look like a badly beaten boxer with puffed up slits for eyes. Next day he was fine. We checked back on his food each time this happened and one day noticed that it was the occasional banana that was the cause. Then we found that even a small piece of banana caused a slight puffiness and some jelly on his eyes. Now he does not eat bananas and he is okay.' The boy's twin does not suffer from this allergy.

## Mouth ulcers

Mary found that in her early forties she suddenly became allergic to cheese. 'I awakened one morning to find my tongue was bright red and sore and I had ulcers on the inside of my mouth. It lasted about six months and was very unpleasant. However I had been eating a lot of cheese and decided eventually to cut it out entirely. Within about two weeks the whole thing had cleared up.' Mary does not eat any cheese now nor yogurt nor anything made of soured milk.

## Headaches and migraine

At least one out of every ten people is thought to be a migraine sufferer. That is a total of over five million people living in Britain. They include all ages, classes, occupations and races.

Migraine is defined by the Migraine Trust as a headache which comes at intervals with complete freedom between attacks. The headache lasts a number of hours and is accompanied by stomach and/or visual symptoms. The stomach symptoms are loss of appetite and the feeling of, or actually being, sick. Constipation often occurs although occasionally sufferers have diarrhoea. Visual disturbances such as flashing lights or an inability to see a certain area may precede an attack and last about 20 to 30 minutes but more commonly there is no warning. During the headache the sufferer will have a dislike of bright lights and many experience difficulty in focusing.

Trials have recently been carried out on children suffering from migraine. Eighty-eight were put on a strict diet after which different foods were introduced. Fifty-five foods were found to cause symptoms which as well as migraine, included stomach pain and diarrhoea, behaviour disorder, aches in limbs, fits, rhinitis (runny nose), mouth ulcers, vaginal discharge, asthma and eczema. Most children reacted to several foods: seventeen to only one and eight to none. Cows' milk, egg, chocolate, orange, wheat, benzoic acid (a preservative, code number E210), cheese, tomato, tartrazine (a food colouring, code number E102) and rye were the worst offenders in that order.[6]

The Migraine Trust does not believe that food is the primary cause of migraine but says certain foods may trigger off attacks in some people. In one recent research project, it was found that many people automatically avoided foods which they thought might cause an attack. Out of 500 people, three-quarters avoided chocolate, nearly half avoided cheese and other dairy products and a quarter gave fruit, particularly citrus fruits, and alcohol a miss. Fifteen per cent avoided tea and coffee. Fried foods, onions and pork were also avoided.[7] In my research chocolate and cheese also appear to cause the most damage although other foods have been thought to be the culprits (see Appendix 3).

Robert discovered chocolate caused his migraine over 35 years ago. He is now 76 years old. He says: 'I suffered from migraine in a very severe form. It stopped me working for a half or whole day: spots in front of my eyes so I could not read, blinding headaches so I could not concentrate at all. This lasted from youth until I was called up in 1941. During those years in the army I hardly suffered at all. But a few weeks after being demobbed it started again. Then I read somewhere that about five different foods could cause migraine – among them chocolate. It was my habit to eat one or two small bars each day. So I stopped eating them and have not had a migraine since. And I still don't eat chocolate.'

Claudia has learned to avoid cheese and coffee. 'I have been a migraine sufferer for many years and although I would not associate every one of these attacks with my diet, I have found that a combination of cheese and coffee, particularly if both are eaten on the same day, guarantee to bring on a severe attack of migraine.'

Carole found that certain meats, chocolate, oranges, cola drinks, cream cheese and the flavour enhancer, monosodium glutamate (621) caused her to have migraine. 'I was put on one after another migraine tablet, none of which worked without making me feel sick. Soon I began to realise that certain foods upset me: feelings of restlessness, yawning, then next day I would have a migraine. I have now learned to avoid these foods with marvellous results.'

There are different kinds of headaches. Enid wrote about hers which she medically termed tri-geminal neuralgia. She discovered, by chance, that it was caused by monosodium glutamate (621). 'I normally work part-time but through pressure of work I was requested to do extra hours so every day for lunch I took a couple of rolls and a flask of packet soup. I started to get neuralgia every day and decided there had to be a clue somewhere. For the first time I read the ingredients on the soup packet. I cut out the soup and lo and behold the neuralgia stopped.' The packet soup had contained monosodium glutamate.

## Hyperactivity

The Hyperactive Children's Support Group claims that possibly one in five children suffers in some form from hyperactivity. It publishes a leaflet which states: 'Many children are hyperactive from birth (they are often so in the womb); they are restless, fidgety, sleep perhaps three to four hours out of 24 and cry almost incessantly. They will not feed properly, whether breast or bottle-fed. No amount of nursing, cuddling or comforting will pacify them.

'As these children grow older, this hyperactive behaviour is accentuated – they seem in a state of perpetual motion which makes them extremely accident prone. Although a high IQ is possible, many hyperactive children experience difficulty in learning. Speech can be a problem and balance is often poor, with extreme clumsiness. They are prone to cot-rocking and head banging; their behaviour is unpredictable and disruptive; they are easily excitable and cry often; they are unable to sit still for more than a few minutes at a time; co-ordination and concentration are very poor.

'They are poor sleepers and eaters. There is often a history of headaches, catarrh, asthma, hayfever and other respiratory complaints; and boys are more likely to be affected than girls. Another strange symptom to emerge is that almost all hyperactive children suffer from acute thirst.

'Mothers feel loners and social outcasts. They feel their children create such havoc wherever they go that they are not welcome in playgrounds, nursery school, shops, friends' or relatives' homes. A simple shopping trip takes on nightmarish qualities.'

The Hyperactive Children's Support Group publishes a handbook which includes the Feingold diet.[8] This diet eliminates certain food additives: artificial colours and flavours, the flavour enhancer monosodium glutamate (621), the benzoate (E210-E219) and nitrate/nitrite (E249-E252) groups of preservatives, and two antioxidants BHA (E320) and BHT (E321). The diet also recommends testing various foods containing salicylate (see p. 76 for a full list) by avoiding and then later reintroducing them individually to see if there is a reaction. The Group says that many children have been helped by this diet.

Linda found the Feingold diet was the answer to her young daughter's problems. 'My daughter who is now four years had never slept through the night until the beginning of the year when my health visitor finally told me about the Feingold diet for hyperactive children. As I was desperate to clutch at any straws, I adopted the diet, kept a diary of food, sleep and behaviour and we are now utterly convinced that Helen is one of those children who is intolerant of salicylates. Thus, the apples, oranges and tomatoes which I had always encouraged, were in fact prime catalysts in causing excessive thirst, waking repeatedly at night and disruptive and aggressive behaviour. Also my daughter cannot tolerate grapes or blackcurrants.'

Margaret's son was also helped by going on the Feingold diet. She says: 'My son, aged 12, has been a constant worry to us. He had terrible behavioural problems. Throughout his life I have tried everything (punishment, extra attention and loving, coaxing and encouragement). Also doctors, psychiatrists and finally a psychologist to assess his concentration level which to us and his teachers was terribly lacking.

'His behaviour was so anti-social that he was disliked by everyone and he was threatened with expulsion by his teachers. Purely by accident we saw Dr Ben Feingold's book on hyperactivity.[8] I was determined to follow his diet. I decided the best way to keep my son on his diet was for all of us to go on it and it has worked very well. My son was a different child within one week – I was amazed. And he has been wonderful keeping to it. My son's psychologist has 'signed him off', agrees the diet has worked and does not want to see him again. Incidentally he did not agree with the diet initially but has come round now. My son's teachers say they have never seen such a difference in a child, almost overnight.

'We have had one or two setbacks when he has eaten a non-permitted food. We have found artificial colouring and flavouring cause serious behavioural problems. Of food with salicylates in them, tomatoes are okay. Raspberries caused depression – he cried for three days.' This may have been because fresh tomatoes are relatively low in salicylates – see p. 76. At the time of writing Margaret had not tested any more foods with salicylates in them to see whether they could be included in her son's diet.

Johanna found additional foods to those mentioned in the Feingold diet caused her daughter problems. These were chocolate and cheese. (Other foods reported to cause hyperactivity are shown in Appendix 3.) Johanna writes. 'My eldest child, now five, has never slept through the night since she was born. She was breast-fed until nine months and has always had a great thirst. When she wakes she has a drink and settles back to sleep. When she was younger a bad night could mean her waking every 15 minutes. I read an article about hyperactivity and although I did not consider her hyperactive, her sleeping behaviour and the drinking seemed to be related.

'I had suspected certain foods caused problems. Orange in any form whether squash, colouring or fruit would mean a bad night with diarrhoea the next morning and if the attack was bad a few patches of eczema. She is also upset by chocolate, other colourings, preservatives, especially in cooked meats, bacon and sausages, tomatoes and cheese. As she has got older her reaction is not so severe. Nights have improved to the point where sometimes she only wakes once or twice on good nights.'

A recent clinical trial[9] on 76 hyperactive children showed that 62 of them improved by eliminating various foods from their diet. Although artificial colouring (tartrazine E102) and preservative (benzoic acid E210) were the commonest provoking substances, no child was sensitive to them alone. Forty-eight different foods were shown to cause trouble with cows' milk, chocolate, grapes, wheat and oranges heading the list.

## Bedwetting and lack of bladder control

Lack of bladder control, whether during the day or at night, creates anxiety in both children and parents. It can be caused by many factors and you should consult your doctor if you are worried about this problem. However if there does not seem to be a physical reason, you may wish to investigate whether a food or drink could be the cause. Here are the stories of two children, a boy and a girl, who suffered for many years with wet pants, until their mothers discovered that what they were eating or drinking was the cause.

Alix's mother discovered that the squash her daughter was drinking was the root of the trouble: 'I started to toilet-train my daughter when she was two years old in the same way as I had successfully trained my son. I was getting nowhere, gave up and put her back in nappies for six months. I then put her back in pants with a few days' success – a few days' failure – and so it went on.

'When she was three and a half I took her to the doctor who said to give her time, that some children gained control earlier than others and not to get anxious. I was concerned but did not relay any anxiety to my daughter. Sometimes she had no control over her bowels either but this was infrequent.

'At four and a half she started school. She took extra pants with her. Needless to say this did not inspire confidence in her but at least there were a few other children with the same problem. It seemed to be getting worse. I waited in vain for her to grow out of it but to no avail.

'At seven years of age I suggested to the doctor that he check for a cause as it did not seem normal. She now had intermittent stomach pain. Apart from the large wash, 40 to 50 pairs of pants, socks, tights etc., per week, Alix was then old enough to realise that "wet pants" did not happen to her friends and consequently she would not play anywhere but at home for fear of an accident.

'Meanwhile she had been to the local hospital for a urine test and examination. Nothing was found amiss. I went back to the doctor as there was now an unusual smell – quite vile – sweet and fishy. By this time I was almost frantic. Arrangements were made for a kidney test at the city hospital. Again nothing could be found.

'The smell persisted and I contacted the doctor at the city hospital and arranged for a mid-stream specimen of urine to be taken. (There were no facilities at the local hospital to analyse this.) An infection was found and a double course of penicillin prescribed. This was terrific and stopped the problem straightaway. The course lasted 20 days and as soon as it was finished she went straight back to the old problem. I tried penicillin again two months later with the same result. This proved to me at least the problem was not physical. I figured that the penicillin was treating the symptoms but not the cause and could not foresee having her on penicillin for long periods.

'I turned then to what she was eating and drinking. I kept a record for a fortnight and then started to eliminate certain food and drink and recording reaction. I finally got it down to "squash". The smell took nearly a week to disappear and within a fortnight she was in control of her bladder and "wee wees" were down to about four per day. She was eight years old. I tried her on squash a few months later with wet pants and smell resulting. She has been fine since.'

One other letter accused squash while another mentioned saccharin in a blackcurrant drink as causing bedwetting. Two more letters cited additives in general as being the culprit. My second example of this type of problem is a boy called Stuart. His mother wrote:

'Stuart is 12 next month and he was three when he started with kidney and bladder problems. Numerous visits to the doctor and several to the hospital told us that something was irritating his bladder but they thought he would grow out of it. At the time he was wetting night and day and did not seem to have any control over his bladder. Over the years daytime control was mastered although Stuart knew he had to move quickly.

'A course of medicine which was supposed to calm the nerves of his bladder had the opposite effect and nearly drove the whole family to the "mad house" as Stuart changed from a contented toddler to an aggressive child. It did not stop the bedwetting.

'At six years the infection stopped. I then decided washing draw sheets was easier than having an upset child and stayed away from the doctor. On hearing a broadcast on local radio we began to wonder if food was the cause. A very bad dose of flu, which laid Stuart flat for a week when he did not eat anything, just drank gallons, decided me for he was dry all week.

'Sugar was suspected because we had always teased Stuart about his sweet tooth. He seemed to have a weight problem and we found, on "dieting" him, there was always an improvement in the bed wetting. I then heard of a place where you send a sample of hair for analysis and it returned saying Stuart was allergic to all forms of sugar. We cut out all foods containing sugar and had an immediate response. I was still allowing him to eat fresh fruit and after a fortnight bedwetting returned but more spasmodically.

'I went "cap in hand" to the doctor to make sure I was not doing any harm cutting out all sugars. She said that as he looked better than she had ever seen him and as it seemed to be working I should continue and write to the local hospital dietician for advice. The sheet they sent tabooed all fresh fruit except cherries and grapes and if we keep to this he is completely dry. Stuart is now much slimmer and full of energy (very lacking before).'

## Stomach upsets

Indigestion, cramps, nausea, vomiting and diarrhoea are stomach ailments which occur from eating a food which does not agree with you. The symptoms can be caused by an inborn or developed deficiency in your body which prevents you metabolizing a particular food, by food poisoning or by plain over-eating. But if you get regular stomach upsets and your doctor is unable to find a satisfactory solution, you should think about whether a particular food or foods may be the cause.

Josephine found she kept on having feelings of nausea which she puts down to eating fish. When she stopped having a light diet consisting of steamed fish every two or three days, she became perfectly all right. She has not eaten fish since then. She thinks this was triggered off by having eaten 'not very fresh prawns'.

Olive suffered from bilious attacks and pinpointed this to eating citrus fruit. She no longer eats any and has found it helpful.

Gloria's teenage daughter started suffering from stomach cramps but the doctor could find nothing physically wrong. 'When she entered her fifth year in school, she decided not to stop for school dinners any more and took brown bread salad sandwiches, yogurt and fruit instead. A few weeks later, I noticed she was not complaining of stomach cramps any more and suggested to her it must have been the cooking at school. Apparently she had decided to take packed lunches because she was bored with the same thing every day. The culprit was the only food she liked on the menu – hot dogs (frankfurters).'

Sylvia's son, aged 15, suffered from periodic bouts of diarrhoea throughout his life and through various trials and her own observations, she tracked it down to certain foods. 'Quite early on, when he was still a toddler, I realised that cola drink was a culprit and have proved that tartrazine (a yellow food colouring, code number E102) is also a cause. Honey is another with the exception of Gales honey.'

## Depression

Depression is a loose term which can describe a variety of feelings and symptoms. Can depression be caused by what you eat? Here are two people who say it can.

For many years Jennifer suffered from bouts of depression, irritability and tiredness. She says: 'Really acute tiredness. I had no grounds for these symptoms. Eventually they started to take hold of my life.' Jennifer went to the doctor and had a thyroid deficiency test which proved negative. She was given a tranquiliser but did not like what it was doing to her. Her doctor then prescribed another. 'This time I burned the prescription when I arrived home.'

She eventually met someone who suggested she have some allergy tests done. She was told she was allergic to all forms of poultry (e.g. chicken, turkey, duck), eggs and to a mild degree, demerara sugar. 'I was convinced it was a con. Anyway I cut out poultry, eggs and demerara sugar from my diet for three months. I felt as if I was reborn. I was 36 at the time but before that I had felt 56. Then after the three months I felt 26 and so happy and so contented. Friends asked what was happening to me. I looked younger, my hair, eyes and skin looked better. It was great to be alive. My husband was amazed.'

Proof of Jennifer's allergy came some time later on a holiday to Guernsey. She was given eggs for breakfast and the following evening duck for dinner. She says: 'The following day – oh, did I feel ill. All the old symptoms were back. Even my aunt asked my husband what was wrong and whatever had made me a Jekyll and Hyde. Needless to say no more eggs or poultry on that holiday. Two and a half years later I find that I can eat poultry once a week and small quantities of egg without problems.'

Anne became depressed after her first baby son was born. She was 25 years old. She writes: 'By the time my son was ten days old I was on a tranquiliser for post-natal depression (the doctor's diagnosis, not mine). Within another two weeks I was an outpatient at the local psychiatric unit and by the time my son was four and a half weeks old I was an in-patient at the unit for the next six months. My story in the unit is much the same as many other psychiatric patients: the doctors have not a clue what to do with you and tell you the illness is all in the mind; you generally feel worse than ever so you just pretend you are well and in the end they discharge you.

'After being discharged I went to stay with my mother for five months, 30 miles away from my home. Therefore I hardly saw my husband for the first year of Stuart's life and Stuart suffered emotional deprivation as I was not well enough to offer love. During the first year I took every different kind of pill and had my mind probed to a great depth. Eventually this led to a nervous breakdown with suicide attempts. Then I saw a succession of private doctors who helped a bit again with medication. However I was far from well. Though my depression had gone, I suffered from continual fatigue which was so bad I tried three times to get Stuart put into care as I was too tired to look after him. I did not succeed.'

Three and a half years after Stuart was born, Anne read a book about allergies and started to eliminate all additives from her diet. As she had felt so tired, she had relied heavily on convenience foods. 'I just could not believe the difference it made. Within a week I felt much more perky. Not only did my continual fatigue disappear, so did insomnia, dreadful nightmares, acne (which I had had for 15 years), the continual need to pass water (once an hour, day and night), vaginal discharge, my periods became regular for the first time in my life, the condition of my hair improved and so the list goes on.'

Anne still feels a slight fatigue in the summer and does not know why. However she does say: 'I think in my case my illness was caused purely through bad diet.' Anne ends her story on a happy note: 'Despite my tale of woe, Stuart has turned out a lovely child. For some reason although I poured rubbish food down my throat, I did not for him. I never gave him sugar or bought him sweets. I always prepared his baby food myself and he never had commercial baby foods. From the day he was born he was a very contented baby. He really is a perfect child.'

## Nightmares

Hugh finds both he and his wife have disturbed sleep with bad dreams and general restlessness if they eat anything with the additive, monosodium glutamate, in it. He says: 'We are convinced that the situation arose from the use of a gravy mix which contains monosodium glutamate (a flavour enhancer, code number 621). In evidence of this, we have noticed that items such as flavoured (not plain) crisps produce the same effect.' Monosodium glutamate is used in most forms and brands of potato crisps except for the plain salted variety.

## Aches, pains and arthritis

There are many forms of arthritis and not all aches and pains are caused by it. The most common forms of arthritis are: osteo-arthritis where the tissues surrounding a joint (e.g. hips, knees and back) start to wear away, becoming narrow and losing their elasticity. And rheumatoid-arthritis when the joints and surrounding tissues become inflamed and swollen. Both types can be extremely painful and disabling, although some people may have quite bad conditions (shown up by X-rays) which do not result in much or any pain.

The medical profession seems unconvinced that the majority of people suffering from arthritic pain can be helped by eliminating certain foods. The official view of the Arthritis and Rheumatism Council is that you should avoid putting on weight, eat a nutritious diet, and if you feel a food does aggravate your arthritis, eliminate it. Dr F. Dudley Hart MD says:[10] 'It is of interest that many patients with osteo or rheumatoid arthritis avoid certain acid foods and drinks as they find symptoms worsen if they take them. Food allergies and idiosyncracies may indeed aggravate arthritic symptoms but these are uncommon as compared with the too rich, too calorie-high diet which, by increasing weight, by decreasing mobility and by diminishing general health, adversely affects all forms of arthritis.'

However, Norman wrote to me saying he had cured himself of both back and hip pain after three days by not eating white flour or anything made with it. Until then he found even walking a strain. He says: 'Most of my adult life, I am now 38, I have been conscious of slight discomfort in my rear pelvis area when standing fully upright. Occasionally I would suffer fairly uncomfortable increases in back pain which I was able to cure with back exercises until a couple of years ago, when I had a recurrence and all the exercises which had previously been successful failed to effect a cure. The pain in my pelvis was so bad I could not walk more than a hundred yards without having to sit down for relief. An X-ray revealed I had a tilted pelvis which had strained the ligaments but the cause of the pain was arthritis in one of the pelvic joints.

'One day a couple of months later I recalled that I had read somewhere previously of a link between arthritis and refined foods. Immediately I stopped eating white bread purchased from a local baker, very nice bread too, and switched back to wholemeal which we had been eating less and less over the previous two years. Within three days my mobility was 95 per cent restored, 100 per cent within a week and has been ever since. Now I am aware only of a slight sensation in that area from time to time, although it is not necessary to have a 100 per cent wholemeal diet. Occasionally I eat white bread. I am now enjoying cricket, basketball and walking again whereas before a visit round to the shops was a severely painful experience.'

Pat found chocolate and eggs affected her badly as well as white flour. She had suffered from swollen and painful ankles and knees and also had bouts of disabling tiredness. She claims that as long as she does not eat these foods, she is completely well. Milk has been reported to have increased one woman's rheumatoid arthritis.[5]

Many different diets have been advocated to relieve the pain of arthritis and several are conflicting. Dr Dong, an American doctor, has written a number of books about arthritis and diet and recommends a diet cutting out all meat, fruit and dairy products as well as some other foods. He says many people suffering from arthritis have been helped by not eating these foods.[11]

Unfortunately Dr Richard Mackarness contradicts certain components of Dr Dong's diet saying that investigations have shown that grain (e.g. wheat), milk, coffee, tea, sugar and pork are the most common foods causing arthritis. He did not find that meat (other than pork) and fruit (other than oranges) caused much problem.[12] Dr Dong's diet allows you to eat wheat, coffee and tea.

This conflicting advice is made worse by another recently published diet for arthritis which says you should fast for three days only drinking orange and lemon juice. It tells you to cut out red meat and eat plenty of whole and unrefined wheat. Who is right? Your guess is as good as mine.

Both Harold and Phyllis followed Dr Dong's diet and found they were much improved. Harold had arthritis in his hands and could not use his fingers. He decided to follow Dr Dong's diet as his doctor only recommended aspirin. He followed the diet strictly for six weeks and found it was pepper and dairy products which caused his trouble. He says this cured him and now has no trouble as long as he does not eat these things.

Phyllis has followed Dr Dong's diet for eight years and finds if she sticks to it she is free of pain, swelling and stiffness. If she deviates, these symptoms return. One of the worst offenders, she finds, is monosodium glutamate (621). She pinpointed this by comparing the effect of different brands of tinned baked beans with and without monosodium glutamate.

One factor which makes it difficult to determine if food might be a cause of arthritis or any aches and pains, is that it can take weeks or even months before any beneficial effect is felt by eliminating certain foods. If this is the case, it is extremely hard to keep up any sort of strict elimination diet unless you are fairly certain of achieving positive results.

## Fits and convulsions

People, especially children, suffering from fits, convlusions and epilepsy *must* seek advice and treatment from their doctor. However, here are two examples of children who were helped dramatically by the elimination of milk and other foods.

Christina was two and a half when her mother wrote to me. Her mother believes the child suffers from an allergy to dairy products which causes convulsions – although this has not been confirmed by the medical profession. 'Christina had her first fits at approximately six months old in exactly the same week that I started weaning her onto cows' milk. This always worried me but to begin with I was told there could be no connection so I put it to the back of my mind. An EEG[13] showed a major brain disturbance although three brain scans have shown no tissue damage. Christina's fits gradually became worse and worse.'

Christina was transferred to a London hospital who were fairly sure she had some degenerative brain disease. Tests were done for every known condition but these all proved negative. 'She was by now having 60 to 70 convulsions a day and had been virtually written off by the hospital as she did not fall into any known diagnosis. However the cows' milk business had remained in my mind and last year I met a number of people who suffered from gastric or skin allergies to dairy produce. I also read an American article on research into other conditions caused by allergy including epilepsy.

'A friend with a skin allergy gave me a diet sheet, told me about soya substitute[14] and suggested I tried a milk-free diet just to put my mind at rest. To our amazement over the next three to four weeks, Christina's fits abated to a dozen or so a week and finally stopped altogether – she has now had none for over a year.

'We have recently weaned her off her anti-convulsant drug and a sedative. These drugs in themselves have held up her progress tremendously although she does have an underlying developmental problem – at the moment she is very much retarded both physically and mentally. We have just begun intensive home therapy.' The hospital has now conceded that Christina is probably not suffering from a degenerative condition and has said it would conduct tests into a possible allergy. Ten months later, when Christina's mother wrote, no tests had been carried out.

Yvonne also found that dairy products caused her daughter, now aged ten, to have fits. From birth this little girl suffered from epilepsy. The fits were more violent when she was small; sometimes she had four to five fits a day. She would throw herself at the wall and become incontinent. At the age of five she started school where she became worse. She was eating school meals. Yvonne's doctor said 'rubbish' to the possibility of food being the cause but when Yvonne saw a specialist he put her daughter on a special diet for a month. She suffered withdrawal symptoms as the specialist had predicted – a continuous fit for 72 hours. After that she was fine. Her daughter cannot eat any dairy products, red food colouring or tea.

In a trial with 88 children suffering from migraine, out of 14 also suffering from fits, 12 stopped having fits when they eliminated certain foods. Two did not improve.[6] In another trial with 76 hyperactive children, of 14 who suffered fits before starting an elimination diet, all but one stopped having fits after excluding certain foods.[9]

Dr J. Egger at Munich University Children's Hospital has recently been conducting tests into whether epilepsy can be caused by specific foods. He has found that only epileptic children suffering from other symptoms such as stomach complaints, migraine or hyperactivity, have shown considerable improvement by manipulating their diet. Children with epilepsy alone have not responded to dietary treatment.

## More than one allergy

Some people suffer from more than one set of symptoms. Many children suffer from eczema as well as asthma. Both these allergies may be related to food, maybe just one; maybe neither. Some doctors feel that if you suffer from more than one allergy, they are more likely to be related to food.

Here is one example of a boy who suffered from three different types of symptoms: eczema, asthma and hyperactivity. His mother writes: 'When Neil was born in 1979 he was never a happy baby. He cried and grizzled a lot and slept very little. He was breast and bottle-fed and when tried on egg had a terrible reaction which frightened me.

'At three months eczema appeared on his feet. As eczema was in my husband's family, I suppose I was not that surprised but I had not realised how aggravating it could be. Sitting up, crawling, walking all happened very quickly. He could still manage without sleep and was so active I could not cope. My doctor had no sympathy and when Neil was two and had not spoken as much as a word, I decided something had to be done as to me he was not normal.

'Asthma was the next thing we had to cope with and he often ended up in hospital. By this time I was very pregnant with my next son and the fact that Neil wheezed and scratched himself from morning till night annoyed me terribly. One morning I read about milk allergies and eczema and asthma and thought what have I got to lose. I started to eliminate cows' milk from his diet and miraculously he got better. Luckily there is a goat farm nearby and I am now able to cater for all his needs.

'However he was still hyperactive. One day I read about additives in foods such as sausages, fish fingers and squash drinks and then it suddenly dawned on me how bad he got after meals. So that day I started him on the purest diet possible. Of course it was not easy, especially struggling along with a limited knowledge of what went into food, but he definitely got better.'

## Notes

1 More information can be obtained from the British Diabetic Association, (address in Appendix 1).
2 Bronchitis is inflammation of the bronchi, the air passages in the lungs; symptoms are similar to asthma.
3 Description provided by the National Eczema Society (address in Appendix 1).
4 *Dietary Treatment of Eczema* prepared by Dr David J. Atherton and Janet Goldsborough, for the National Eczema Society, 1983.
5 *Food Intolerance and Food Aversion,* a joint report of the Royal College of Physicians and the British Nutrition Foundation, April 1984.
6 *Is Migraine Food Allergy?,* J. Egger et al, The Lancet, 15 October 1983.
7 *Understanding Migraine,* Migraine Trust.
8 The Feingold diet originates from Dr Ben Feingold's book *Why Your Child is Hyperactive,* Random House, New York, 1975. The Hyperactive Children's Support Group's handbook costs £3 (see Appendix 1 for address).
9 *Controlled Trial of Oligoantigenic Treatment in the Hyperkinetic Syndrome,* J. Egger et al, The Lancet, 9 March 1985.
10 *Diet and Arthritis,* F. Dudley Hart MD, published in Arthritis and Rheumatism Council Magazine No 56, Summer 1983.
11 *New Hope for the Arthritic,* Colin H. Dong MD and Jane Banks, Hart Davis, MacGibbon.
12 *Chemical Victims,* Dr Richard Mackarness, Pan Books, 1980.
13 An EEG is an electro-encephalogram which records electrical impulses in the brain.
14 Soya milk is an alternative to cows' milk: see p. 154. Goats' and sheep's milk may also be suitable alternatives: see Chapter 6.

# 3

# How to find the cause

If you suspect that a food or drink is causing your, or your child's, allergy how do you find out which one? Most people eat a vast range of food and drink. How can you pinpoint which food or foods are causing the damage? It probably seems like a tangled ball of wool which you have no hope of unravelling; a needle in a haystack.

One lady told me she was totally confused after a visit to a hospital doctor. She had consulted him in a bid to help her eczema. He had told her not to eat food with colouring in it and had given her two lists which she claimed were contradictory. She was young and intelligent, a literary agent used to dealing with the written word but she felt at a total loss to know what to do.

There are several ways to start your search for a food culprit. The simplest, and a very constructive way, is to keep a diary: a record of everything you eat and drink and what your symptoms have been.

## Keep a diary

I discovered the foods which caused my son's allergies by this simple method. It only involved myself. For several years my son did not even know I was keeping a record. I kept a diary of everything he ate and how he was each day. This way I was able to see if any pattern emerged between his health and what he ate. Was he ill after eating a certain food? Did this happen every time or did he sometimes eat that food with no ill effect? How long after eating the suspect food did the reaction occur? And how long did the symptoms last? By keeping a diary you will be doing something positive to discover if the reason for your allergy is a food. And it should enable you to discover which foods can be eaten as well as those which should be avoided. It will also cause the minimum inconvenience to yourself and the rest of your family.

This is how to do it: keep two diaries. One should contain how the sufferer was and felt and include any medicine taken; the other should contain everything he or she ate and drank. The diaries should be pocket-sized but have enough space to enter full details. I use two separate diaries as most small diaries do not contain enough space for both sets of information to be clearly entered. A single, larger, office-style diary may be sufficient to take details of both food and symptoms but should not be so big as to be a bother to carry about if you need to take it on holiday or away for any reason. The two sets of information should be detailed in separate columns: this way you will find it easier to refer to as all the information is not jumbled together.

Fill in your diaries at least once a day. I found the best time was in the evening before going to bed but you may well find another time more convenient. Make it a regular habit, like brushing your teeth, and you will soon find it easy to do. It should only take about five minutes each day. The importance of keeping a diary is that it is impossible to remember what you or your child has eaten or felt even a week ago. This way you will have exact details in writing. Try and remember what you ate for lunch this day last week or three weeks ago. You most probably cannot.

It is important to keep up the diaries even when you, or your child, are going through a good period. It is all too easy to say 'I am all right now' and stop recording. However you may suddenly go through a bad patch and then it is very useful to refer back to see if certain foods or groups of foods eaten together gave you any trouble during the good time. If you were okay eating them during your good period, you can be pretty sure they are not the cause of your symptoms during your bad patch.

## 'How you are' diary

This should contain:
• How the sufferer felt that day (morning, afternoon, evening and night): list all symptoms e.g. wheezing, eczema on face, tearful or disruptive mood, okay or clear (no symptoms); and how bad they were e.g. slight, bad, terrible. It may not be possible to record all of a child's symptoms as you will probably not know how he or she was at school; unless of course they were bad enough for the teacher to tell you or ask for the child to be taken home.

• Did the sufferer need medicine to relieve the symptoms: what medicine, how much and at what time?
   Note these if you feel they are relevant:

• Mood changes e.g. bad, good, high (excitable), low (depressed). If you are charting the health of a hyperactive child, for instance, you will want to note mood changes in detail every day. However where this is not specifically the problem, you may still find it useful to note any extreme mood changes.

• The weather: hot, dry, humid, cold, raining. Often damp weather can bring on aches and pains and it may be interesting to discover whether there really is a connection between that rainy day and your backache. Also a sudden change in weather conditions or drop or rise in pressure (on a barometer) may be significant.

• An accurate grass pollen count; and plants, trees or flowers which are budding or blooming (see p. 85).

• Whether windows were open or closed.

• Smell of rubber or plastic in room or house caused by books, toys, balloons, or fumes caused by cooking, frying, gas or paint.

• Change of environment e.g. on holiday at relatives' home.

• Encounter with animals you don't usually meet e.g. cat in friend's home.

• Change of toiletries e.g. soap, deodorant, perfume, toothpaste, make-up, washing powder.

**Example of 'How you are' diary**

---

## April 1984                        am

| Sun | 1 | *Clear* |
|------|-----|---------|
| Mon | 2 | *Clear (on plane)* |
| Tues | 3 | *Hot   Clear* |
| Wed | 4 | *Rain  clear* |
| Thur | 5 | *Sunny wheezy  Ⓟ 8·30 Ⓥ 9·30 Ⓟ 11·30* |
| Fri | 6 | *Sunny wheezy   Ⓟ 9·30 Ⓟ 11·30* |
| Sat | 7 | *Sunny wheezy* |
| Sun | 8 | *Sunny bit wheezy* |
| Mon | 9 | *Rain   clear* |
| Tues | 10 | *Sunny   clear* |
| Wed | 11 | *Sun/cloud clear* |
| Thur | 12 | *Sun/cloud clear* |
| Fri | 13 | *Cloudy   clear* |
| Sat | 14 | *Cloudy   clear* |
| Sun | 15 | *Cloudy   clear* |

Abbreviations are as follows: P stands for a homoeopathic pill; V stands for Ventolin. The numbers refer to the time the medicine was given.

**pm**                    **April 1984**

Clear
Clear
Clear

8pm   Slight wheeze

(P) 1·30   (P) 4·30   (V) 7·40

(V) 5 very wheezy   (V) 11·45

(V) 3·30   (V) 7·00

Clear
Clear
Clear
Clear
Clear
Clear
Clear
Clear

## 'Food and drink' diary

This should contain details of everything the sufferer eats and drinks. There should be enough space each day to include breakfast, lunch, tea, supper and any snacks in between. Abbreviate words as much as possible but remember you need to be able to read them a few weeks later. Here are a few examples but you will soon make up your own: B breakfast, L lunch, T tea, S supper; bd bread, mk milk, choc chocolate, jc juice, squ squash; w white, b brown.

Remember to note down everything including sweets and drinks. Detail flavours and brands of processed foods. It is not sufficient to write just 'ice cream' or 'jam'; you must note the flavour and even the ingredients of these as they can vary between manufacturers. Keep and date the labels if you do not record individual ingredients. You can then refer to them when necessary.

## A child's diaries

Keeping your child's diaries may be slightly more complicated than if you are making notes about your own health. You may not know how your child felt or behaved during school hours for example; although if you confide in your child's teacher, you may well find the school extremely helpful.

You will also have less control over your child's eating habits. If your child is under five and not at school, you should still try and find out what has been eaten when he or she is not with you, on a visit to friends or relatives, for instance. The child may be eating things you do not normally give.

You have two ways of dealing with these situations. You may allow your child to eat and drink whatever he or she likes and check afterwards with the host what has been eaten. Alternatively you may mention beforehand what the child should not be eating. This can be difficult if the host is not aware of what goes into food. She may not suspect, for example, that her fish fingers and squash drink contain colouring or that crisps and sausages have flavour enhancer added to them. The best thing to do is to mention to the host the obvious foods and drinks to avoid and check afterwards exactly what your child has eaten and drunk. Try to avoid making your child's host feel unhappy or uncomfortable about having your child. Explain the position and your child's allergy. It will help your host understand and co-operate. If you do not, it might put off your friend or relative asking your child again which would be a shame. Your child will miss out on forming new relationships and you, maybe, a well earned rest!

A child attending school will encounter more problems. If your child must eat school dinners, this is the greatest problem as school meals contain additives of all sorts and are made up of a combination of many foods. If you can, send your child to school with a packed lunch instead. This is by far the best way of avoiding trouble. Even so, you must also be aware that your child may still be eating foods at school you do not know about. Drinks and cake given to celebrate a child's birthday, shared crisps and other snacks between friends must all be considered.

## Discovering the cause

After you have kept your diaries for some weeks, start to analyse what has been happening. If you are allergic to only one or two foods, which are not eaten very frequently, these offenders will soon become apparent. You will notice that only when you have eaten these foods, will you have a reaction but you are clear the rest of the time. The reaction might start almost immediately after you have eaten the food or up to 24 hours afterwards, possibly after an even longer period; although the longer the delay, the more difficult it is to tie down the cause. Drinks tend to 'show' themselves more quickly than foods which take longer to be digested. Reactions can last for up to four days and maybe longer.

Before you decide that a particular food is the cause, check whether you have eaten it and been okay for the following couple of days. If you have eaten it and had no symptoms, it is probably not the cause although if it was eaten with another food and these two regularly preceded an attack, or if you have eaten more of it than usual, you may have made a discovery.

## Example of 'Food and drink' diary

# April 1984

**2   Monday**   *B- Weetabix / Milk.*
*L- Cheese chips (ok) / marmite / butter / white bread / apple / water.*
*S- Poached egg / wholemeal toast / Danish cheese / water.*

**3   Tuesday**   *B- Weetabix / milk.*
*L- Chicken / lettuce / onion / tomato / oil + vinegar / 7up / strawberries / onion roll / butter.*
*S- Salad / cod / lemon juice / white bread / butter / water.*

**4   Wednesday**   *B- Weetabix / milk.*
*L- Scallops fried / butter garlic / waffle / maple syrup / 7up (Restaurant).*
*S- White toast / bottled fish (ok) / lettuce / mayonnaise / strawberries*

**5   Thursday**   *B- Weetabix / milk.*
*L- Mozarella cheese / wholemeal toast / Danish cheese / 7up.*
*S. Chicken (no salt) / strawberries / 7up.*

**6   Friday**   *B- Weetabix / milk.*
*L- Chicken / white toast / lettuce / 7up / mayonnaise.*
*S- Scallops (at home) / garlic / butter / 7up.*

**7   Saturday**   *B- Weetabix / milk / tea.*
*L- Beefburger (home) / roll / 7up / strawberries.*
*S- Plaice (no seasoning) / mixed salad (no dressing) white bread (Buccaneer Restaurant)*

**8   Sunday**   *B- Weetabix / milk.*
*L- Beefburger (home) / barbecue sauce (ok) / salad / strawberries.*
*S- Crab / avacado / melon / white toast / butter / strawberries.*

The abbreviation (OK) means the ingredients have previously been proved to be safe; (home) means home made; (ketchup) means Heinz tomato ketchup.

# April 1984

**9 Monday**    B- Weetabix / milk.
L- 2 egg omelette / onion / garlic / white toast / butter / lettuce /
   tomato / mayonnaise / olives (ok) / sunflower oil.
S- chicken / barbecue sauce (ok) / 7up / lemon yogurt (ok)
   wholemeal toast / butter walnuts.

**10 Tuesday**    B- Weetabix / milk.
L- Mozarella cheese / wholemeal bread / onions / tomato
   ketchup (ok) / 7up / Danish cheese / apple.
S- Beefburger (home) / barbecue sauce (ok) / roll / onion / mustard /
   7up / strawberries / almond ice cream (ok) / lettuce / tomato.

**11 Wednesday**    B- Weetabix / milk.    L- 2 egg omelette /
onion / garlic / sunflower oil / 7up / wholemeal toast /
lettuce / vinegar / strawberries / cheese straws (ok).
S- Beefburger / roll / ketchup (ok) / mustard / onion / 7up / lettuce
tomato / sunflower oil / vinegar / strawberries / rich tea biscuit.

**12 Thursday**    B- Weetabix / milk.
L- chicken / barbecue sauce / 7up / white toast / butter /
   grapefruit.          T- biscuits (ok).
S- mixed salad / plaice (no seasoning) / 7up / white bread.

**13 Friday**    B- Weetabix / milk.
L- wholemeal bread / Danish cheese / lettuce / 7up /
   strawberries / cheese sticks (ok).
S- Beefburger (home) / roll / ketchup / mustard / onion /
   strawberries / 7up.

**14 Saturday**    B- Rice crispies / milk / tea.
L- chicken / lettuce / tomato / oil + vinegar.
S- Beefburger (home) / roll / onion / mustard / ketchup /
   7up / strawberries / melon.

**15 Sunday**    B- Weetabix / milk.
L- Beefburger (home) / roll / ketchup / mustard / 7up /
   strawberries.
S- Toast / Danish cheese / butter / rice crispies / milk.

Some entries refer to mixed salad; this is because the ingredients did
not affect my son. If you are beginning your search you should list
every ingredient.

## Charting your allergy

A good way of seeing if any pattern emerges between your symptoms and what you eat is by making a chart of all the information you have collected from your diaries. This may seem complicated to start with but it is well worth the time (a couple of hours a month) you spend on it. See my example opposite as a guide.

You will need a piece of graph paper and a pencil (and rubber for easy correction). The graph paper should be large enough (A4 or foolscap size) to chart a whole month (31 days). Use each main division box along the bottom row as a day. Write in the year, month, day and M for Monday, Tu for Tuesday and so on. Leave enough space (about 2 in. on the left) to write in the foods to be analysed. Alternatively you can buy sheets of the *Allergy? Think About Food Chart*.[1]

Decide on grades of how you or your child feel. With my son, I blacked in one main vertical square for wheezing which did not need medicine, two if he needed one dose of medicine that day, three if he needed two doses and so on. If you do not take medicine, you may want to grade your symptoms according to their

---

On the right I have charted my son's condition for the period of 1–17 April 1984. At the bottom of the chart is a record of whether he had any symptoms, and how acute they were, measured by the amount of medicine he took. As he took two sorts of medicine, I have counted two doses of the shorter acting one as equal to one dose of the longer acting one. At the top of the chart is a record of some of the food he ate on each of the days. Almost all the foods were eaten on days when no symptoms appeared, as well as during the attack. Therefore they could not be the cause. I believe the attack was brought on by the scallops eaten at lunchtime on Wednesday 4 April in a restaurant. As scallops were also eaten at home on 6 April when the attack was subsiding, the scallops themselves were not to blame. The cause was probably monosodium glutamate added to the seasoning. But it could have been some ingredient of the waffle, to which he is not normally allergic.

# Example of a food allergy chart

| Food | 1 | 2 | 3 | 4 | 5 | 6 | 7 | 8 | 9 | 10 | 11 | 12 | 13 | 14 | 15 |
|---|---|---|---|---|---|---|---|---|---|---|---|---|---|---|---|
| Waffle | | | | X | | | | | | | | | | | |
| Scallops | | | | X | | X | | | | | | | | | |
| Tomato | | | X | | | X | X | X | X | X | X | X | X | X | X |
| Danish Cheese | | X | | | X | | | | X | | | X | | X | X |
| Egg | | X | | | | | | X | X | | | | | | |
| Beef | X | | | | | X | X | | X | X | | X | X | X | X |
| Chicken | | | X | | X | X | | | X | | | X | | X | |
| Strawberries | | | X | X | X | | X | X | | X | X | | X | X | X |
| Milk | X | X | X | X | X | X | X | X | X | X | X | X | X | X | X |
| Weetabix | X | X | X | X | X | X | X | X | X | X | X | ✱ | X | | X |

(Waffle and Scallops day 4 marked **RESTAURANT**; Scallops day 6 marked **HOME**)

| SYMPTOM OR MEDICINE CHART | | 1 | 2 | 3 | 4 | 5 | 6 | 7 | 8 | 9 | 10 | 11 | 12 | 13 | 14 | 15 |
|---|---|---|---|---|---|---|---|---|---|---|---|---|---|---|---|---|
| | If Medicine taken | | | | | | | | | | | | | | | |
| | 6 DOSES | | | | | | | | | | | | | | | |
| | 5 DOSES | | | | | | | | | | | | | | | |
| If no Medicine taken | 4 DOSES | | | | | | | | | | | | | | | |
| | 3 DOSES | | | | | | | | | | | | | | | |
| TERRIBLE | 2 DOSES | | | | | | | | | | | | | | | |
| BAD | 1 DOSE | | | | | | | | | | | | | | | |
| SLIGHT | SLIGHT | | | | | | | | | | | | | | | |
| Month APRIL   Year 1984 | | 1 | 2 | 3 | 4 | 5 | 6 | 7 | 8 | 9 | 10 | 11 | 12 | 13 | 14 | 15 |
| Fill in day, e.g. M. Tu. W. Th. F. Sa. Su. | | Su | M | Tu | W | Th | F | Sa | Su | M | Tu | W | Th | F | Sa | Su |

intensity e.g. for slight symptoms use one blacked square, for bad symptoms use two, and if terrrible use three squares.

Then, list down the left-hand side of the chart all the foods (or anything else) you suspect and put a mark (cross or circle) above the date when they were eaten. You can then see not only if a food was eaten and caused a reaction but also if it was eaten and did *not* cause any trouble. If the food could be eaten and no reaction occurred or if it was eaten at the end of a bad time and the beginning of a good patch, you can be pretty sure this food is not to blame and can be considered 'safe'. Charting your allergy in this way may seem difficult and time-consuming at first but it can be extremely rewarding when a food is isolated. You will have proof if the food is eaten again and a reaction occurs.

By keeping this chart you may more easily observe if your symptoms occur at specific times of the month or every so often. You may notice that your symptoms take on a similar pictorial pattern. In the example shown you will notice an escarpment shape: a mountain rising sharply on the first day and then gradually descending over the next two days or so. This is for my son a typical food reaction shape. However if the black boxes remain the same height for a few days and a suspect food has not been eaten continually during the period, this signifies to me that the cause of his wheezing is more likely to be an airborne irritant.

## Suspect everything

What should you do if the allergy is continuing every day and there is no clear pattern? Try and think back to when you or your child were going through a better period. Was there a particular food or drink which was *not* eaten or drunk which now is? If you suspect a food or drink, eliminate it from your diet. Then see if you get better. With most allergies an improvement should occur within a few days. If the food is one which you eat regularly, it could happen that you feel worse before you feel better. But avoid it for at least three weeks.

But what if you cannot think of any particular food? Or this does not work? Do not despair: use the following guidelines.

## Keep a 'safe' food list

Note down all the foods which you have been able to eat with no symptoms during the following two or three days. You can consider these foods 'safe' and use them alongside foods you will want to test out. Add to this list as you continue your research.

## Eliminate additives

First, eliminate all colourings, flavourings, flavour enhancers, antioxidants and as many preservatives and other additives as is possible. The worst offenders are described in Chapter 10. More information on individual additives is given in Appendix 2. You will have to study labels on packaging in your local shop or supermarket to discover which foods contain these additives and it will take you longer to do your shopping at first. However you will soon learn what to avoid and what can be eaten. See Chapter 4 for information on labelling.

You may at this stage be saying to yourself 'What on earth do I eat or give to my child if I have to cut all this out?' Do not worry, you will find plenty.

You will find plain fish in the freezer compartment at the supermarket alongside fish that is coated with coloured breadcrumbs. Grill, steam or fry with a bit of butter or vegetable oil and perhaps a pinch of salt and pepper, or better still a herb or two. It will taste just as good and takes no more time. Alternatively you can make your own batter.

Fresh mince bought from your butcher will produce just as good a hamburger as frozen ones containing preservatives and a flavour enhancer. Just add a little salt or pepper and maybe some chopped onion.

Plain yogurt mixed with fresh fruit and perhaps a little sugar must surely be as delicious as those bright, artificially coloured varieties sold in Britain. Fruit yogurts without any additives are beginning to appear in the shops. Look out for them.

You can find plain salted potato crisps amongst the many others using a flavour enhancer, and perhaps colouring. Get your kids to eat them instead. Plain salted crisps may contain an antioxidant. Be aware of this fact.

Grilled meat and fish, fresh vegetables, fruit and nuts, eggs, milk and most cheese all make good quick nutritious meals free from additives. These are just a few examples. I am sure you will think of many more. Avoid using coloured toothpaste and any drugs or medicated sweets which contain colours or additives you suspect. See Chapter 12 for information on medicines and toothpaste.

## Eliminate individual foods

If after a few weeks there is no improvement, you must look to individual foods which may be causing the allergy. The most common foods which cause allergies are: cows' milk and this includes all dairy produce like butter, cream, yogurt and cheese; wheat which includes bread, pastry and breakfast cereals; and eggs. Chocolate, oranges, coffee, peanuts, beef, chicken and sugar are also known to cause trouble but in my research I have found there are many other foods which can trigger off symptoms. I have given examples throughout this book and give more examples of individual foods causing allergies in Chapters 5 to 9. In recent trials involving children suffering from migraine, 55 different foods were shown to cause reactions in one or more of them. Other symptoms such as stomach complaints, behaviour disorder and aches in limbs were also provoked.[2]

Begin by cutting out one food or group of foods. Remember you should consider not only the food in its natural state but you should also check that it is not mentioned in the list of ingredients of bought, processed food. For instance milk goes into chocolate, many margarines in the form of whey, into some bread and rolls as milk or whey powder, and in many canned foods (possibly described as casein or caseinate), as well as ordinary dairy produce; wheat also goes into many tinned and bottled foods in the form of starch as well as in bread, rolls, spaghetti, biscuits, pastries, cakes and breakfast cereals. More details in Chapters 6 and 7.

Avoid the food or group of foods for at least three weeks. Occasionally people suffer withdrawal symptoms at the beginning, that is they get worse before they get better, but these should only last for a couple of days, or possibly a bit longer.Withdrawal symptoms from coffee are particularly well known.

As well as cutting out one particular food, vary the rest of your diet: avoid eating the same food every day for long periods. Leave five days, preferably a week, between eating the same food if you suspect it but do not want to cut it out completely.

At the end of the month, study your diary and chart carefully. Have you been clear of symptoms? If not, see if any of the foods you have been eating could be the culprit.

If you reintroduce the food you have avoided eating, see if you react to it. This should be a pretty good test as to whether that food is in fact a cause. Eat only a small amount to begin with as some people have been known to get a very strong reaction after reintroducing a food. Eat it with foods you feel are 'safe' (those foods you have eaten through a symptom-free period). If you do not react after you have eaten it a few times, add the food to your 'safe' list.

If you have no success eliminating one group after a month, try another. That is what Sue did. Her son Paul, aged five, had suffered from eczema since he was five months old. She was told it was in the family as both her mother and mother-in-law suffered from asthma. Sue wrote: 'By the time Paul was three years old, I noticed that sometimes the eczema was bad and other times he hardly had any. Someone suggested to me he might be allergic to cows' milk as I changed from powdered milk to cows' milk when he was five months old and he also went onto solids at that time.

'I put him onto goats' milk for five weeks and nothing happened. So I decided it might be something else he was eating. I kept a note of everything he ate for four weeks, even what sweets he ate and noted down when the eczema was worse. Sure enough there was a definite pattern. Every time he ate pastry, pies, cakes etc., it was worse. So I presume he is allergic to flour. I can most often now control his eczema by making sure he only eats pastry when his skin is clear. I let him have some now and then because he loves cakes and sausage rolls.'

Sue discovered this two years ago. Unfortunately Paul is not completely clear of his eczema and recently it has flared up again.

Sue will have to investigate further to find the cause. However she noticed a pattern by keeping a diary of how Paul was and found she could improve his condition by cutting out pastry for most of the time. She also discovered that milk was not causing his eczema.

Do not be afraid to make a guess at which food or ingredient might be causing the trouble. There is no harm in eliminating it for a short time to see if you or your child improves by not eating it, but make sure your child eats enough other foods to compensate for any vitamin or mineral deficiency (see Chapter 13).

## What if you are allergic to many foods?

If you feel you can sensibly eliminate more foods from your diet in order to test them, do so but consider the dangers and trouble involved. When Dr Egger and his colleagues discovered the foods which caused the children in their research project to suffer from migraine, the children went onto a very basic diet of one meat (lamb or chicken), one carbohydrate (rice or potato), one fruit (banana or apple), one vegetable (brassica, e.g., cauliflower, cabbage) water and vitamin supplements. The children were kept on this diet for one month to see whether either of the food alternatives was acceptable and no symptoms occurred. Then individual foods were reintroduced once a week.

However Dr Egger's report does stress: 'Diets are dangerous and socially disruptive so such treatment should be adopted only when the symptoms are severe and only under experienced medical and dietetic supervision.'

If you are an adult sufferer and feel you can sustain this kind of diet, you may wish to give it a try. But if you are dealing with a child, you should think very carefully before embarking on such a strict diet. If you do wish to go ahead, you must ask your doctor to help you and seek advice from your local hospital or community dietician (at some hospitals you can approach the dietician direct). A dietician can advise you on diet and whether you need extra vitamins or minerals during this time. Remember that vitamin or mineral supplements should not be coloured or contain any additives or ingredients which may affect you. If necessary, check with the manufacturer what they contain. Bio-Health supplements do not contain any additives (address in Appendix 1).

Be cautious about going on a very strict elimination diet. It can cause a lot of bother and disturbance to you and your family. To live on a diet where many foods are not allowed, even for a few weeks, may be too difficult for most people and for some unnecessary. To be confined to such a diet when the rest of the family are eating many foods must be incredibly hard and for a child almost unbearable. It is bad enough when only a few foods are excluded but when there are so many, life can become intolerable. Where children are concerned, it will be almost impossible to enforce, especially if the child is at school. Even if he or she takes lunch to school, the temptations of a friend's lunch box may be too hard to resist.

If you can discover the food culprits by less severe means, you will be making life a lot easier for yourself. Remember cutting out foods with additives can do no harm at all as long as the equivalent foods are eaten without them. Cutting out one food and its group, or possibly a few individual foods, will also do no harm as long as sufficient nutritious foods are eaten to compensate.

## Special diets

Several diets are now published which either recommend you to eat or tell you to avoid certain foods. Some are aimed at specific conditions, e.g. hyperactivity in children, or come as part of a larger package of help to certain sufferers, for instance sufferers from eczema. Self-help groups giving additional advice in their particular field are listed in Appendix 1.

However, many diets seem contradictory and confusing. For instance some diets exclude wheat whilst others include it. The same may apply to sugar or coffee and tea. As shown in the section on arthritis on p. 52, there are two diets claiming to help sufferers: one says eat fruit, the other says don't. Diets often fall into the meat or vegetarian category: the meat and fish diet which tells you to eat these and excludes wheat and other grains; and the vegetarian diet which eliminates meat but encourages the eating of grains and vegetables.

Some diets are called 'rotated' diets which involve eating certain foods on certain days for a number of weeks. Each food must be eaten only once every four to seven days. Often a fast is recommended before the diet is commenced. These diets are complicated and difficult to sustain.

Ignore all these diets until you have tried my method first. My research has shown that almost any food can cause a reaction so go by your diary, record all you eat and drink and any symptoms and see if a pattern emerges. This is an easier and far less worrying way of starting to discover if food is a cause of your allergy. Most people, on being given so much difficult or conflicting advice, quite rightly 'turn off', lift their hands in horror and say 'I can't possibly get to the bottom of this.' Follow my guidelines. It helped me and others; it can help you.

## Related food

In many books about allergies you will find lists of 'food families'. These food families are based on botanical categories: for example the grass family consists of wheat, rye, barley, oats, corn, rice and sugar cane; and the apple family consists of apples, pears and quince. From these categories you might assume that if you are allergic to one member of the food family e.g. wheat, you are likely to be allergic to another member of the same family e.g. corn or rice. I have found little evidence to support this from my own survey and Dr Egger, who conducted food allergy trials with children who suffered from migraine and hyperactivity, agrees. He found no connection of food allergy within a food family with the exception of citrus fruit (e.g. orange, grapefruit, lemon, lime, tangerine and satsuma). He even complained that this was a pity as a connection would have made his job much easier.

Food, like everything else on this planet, is made up of a variety of natural chemical components. It could be a specific chemical or group of chemicals in certain foods which triggers off your allergy and these foods may not be in the same botanical family. Listed below are some substances which link foods in this way. There is controversy over whether these substances are the common cause of symptoms. So I recommend that you consider and test each food separately.

**Caffeine** is a natural component of coffee, tea, cocoa (chocolate) and cola nuts. There is more caffeine in coffee than in tea – but it depends on how strong you make them. As a rough guide, a cup of coffee contains about 70 mg, a cup of tea about 40 mg. A can of cola drink contains about 30 mg and one ounce of dark chocolate (half a small bar) about 20 mg. Caffeine is added to some pain-killers, drugs for migraine and certain cold and 'flu remedies as well as some soft fizzy drinks.

Caffeine is a stimulant and can be addictive: many coffee drinkers are hooked on it and would get withdrawal symptoms such as a headache or tiredness if they suddenly stopped drinking it. In a recent report[3] the Royal College of Physicians states that caffeine can cause headaches and migraine and that large doses of both coffee and tea can produce nausea and vomiting in susceptible subjects.

From my survey, 35 people said that either coffee or chocolate affected them badly but only seven of these said they could not consume both and just one lady pointed out that she could not drink tea as well as coffee. If you can tolerate one of these foods or drinks and not another, this would indicate that it is not the caffeine in these foods which is the cause of the trouble.

**Gluten** is a mixture of proteins found in wheat and rye; to a lesser extent in oats and barley. Six people wrote saying gluten caused symptoms. But of 16 others who said they could not eat wheat, only one included oats, rye and barley. Only one lady mentioned oats alone caused her asthma.

People with coeliac disease are advised by doctors to avoid gluten. Some multiple sclerosis sufferers do not eat anything containing it either, although there is medical disagreement over the link between this disease and the food. Elizabeth was diagnosed as a coeliac sufferer in 1976, put on a gluten-free diet and then discovered that gluten had also caused her migraine. 'From that day on I have not had one attack of migraine. It could not have worked by suggestion as I had no idea there could be any connection.'

Dr Egger, who conducted tests which showed that children suffering from migraine and hyperactivity reacted to certain foods, says that he found gluten was probably not the factor responsible for a reaction as 50% of the children who could not eat wheat, could in fact tolerate rye.

**Histamine** is a substance found in your body. Usually only a small amount is present but high levels have been discovered in the saliva of asthma sufferers and in the skin conditions of many people. It is also thought to be a cause of migraine. Foods kept for a long time like cheese, salami and canned fish contain a lot of histamine. Foods thought to be histamine-releasers are: egg white, shellfish, strawberries, tomatoes, chocolate, fish, pork, pineapple, pawpaw and alcohol.[4] If you feel histamine is the cause of your allergy, you may care to test the validity of this grouping for yourself.

**Salicylate** is a substance found in aspirin and aspirin is known to cause allergic reactions such as skin rashes, hayfever or asthma.[5] If you are allergic to aspirin, you may be allergic to certain foods which contain salicylate. Recent research in Australia has revealed that many foods contain salicylate.[13] Most fruit contain significant amounts with dried fruit like sultanas, raisins, prunes and figs having higher levels. All berries contain it but amounts vary: raspberries contain four times as much as strawberries according to the survey. Even different varieties of apple vary – Granny Smith apples contain seven times as much as Golden Delicious which have very little. Other fruit containing some are apricots, avocados, blackberries, cherries, black and red currants, cranberries, dates, grapes, grapefruit, loganberries, mandarins, melons, nectarines, oranges, peaches and pineapple. Fruit not mentioned here are likely to contain less (apart from berries). Those containing very little are bananas, pears and lemons plus exotic fruit such as mango and passion fruit.

Vegetables contain less salicylate than fruit. Broccoli, cucumber, endive, radishes and courgettes contain more than other vegetables and canned gherkins, mushrooms and green olives have considerable amounts. Tomatoes contain very little but tomato paste, soup and sauce have more. Some spices and herbs such as curry, paprika, thyme and rosemary contain a lot. So does Worcestershire sauce.

Tea contains significantly more than coffee. Cocoa and carob have none. Nuts differ considerably with almonds and peanuts having the most. Honey again varies considerably between different brands. Cereals (with the exception of maize), fish, meat and dairy produce contain very little or none.

Synthetic salicylate is used to flavour sweets, ice-cream, soft drinks and cake mixes.[3]

There is considerable controversy as to whether salicylate can cause problems in hyperactive children. Dr Feingold found that by eliminating about 20 foods containing salicylate, children suffering from hyperactivity improved.[6] Other researchers claim to have refuted Feingold's results[3] and in 1985 a trial with 76 hyperactive children showed that salicylate was not thought to be a cause as some foods containing salicylate, e.g. peaches and cucumber, produced reactions in very few children.[7] However research in Australia came up with different results.[12] In an investigation of 86 children suffering from behaviour problems, three-quarters reacted to salicylate. The researchers carrying out this project say 'Adverse reactions occur when the dose threshold is exceeded, and depend on the amount consumed and frequency, as well as on recent intake of other foods containing the same compound.' So you may be able to eat individual foods containing salicylate but if you eat too many or too much, you may begin to react.

**Tyramine** is a chemical which can cause headaches and urticaria (a rash). Cheese, especially mature and blue veined cheese, canned and bottled fish, and yeast extract products like Marmite, Bovril and Oxo contain significant amounts. So to a lesser extent do red wine, beer, avocado pears, oranges, bananas, red plums and tomatoes. Chocolate and broad beans contain similar substances which can also cause headaches.[4] Other foods containing these substances are peanuts and other nuts, pork, bacon, ham, pineapple and grapes.[12]

## Combination of foods

You may find that it is only a combination of certain foods which triggers off your allergy. Liz found that tea and Marmite consumed at the same time made her feel sick and headachy. Vanilla and orange; egg cooked with butter; coffee and cheese taken together: all were given as examples of combinations causing trouble to individuals. After you have kept your diary for a while, you may spot a common link.

## Tolerance levels

Some people may react violently to only a tiny portion of food to which they are allergic. A small amount can trigger off an attack lasting several days. That is why it is important to note down in your diary all that you have eaten. You may discover that it is a small ingredient in a food rather than the main one which is the cause and common factor between different foods. For example, milk, eggs, wheat and sugar are ingredients of many recipes (both shop and home-made) and additives such as colouring, preservative and flavouring, go into many different processed foods. Only a small amount may be used but this can still cause a reaction.

Other sufferers may be able to tolerate a certain amount; or be able to eat a cooked food but not that food in its raw state. Dorothy suffered for many years with sick headaches until she discovered that cheese, chocolate and eggs were the cause. She says she hardly ever has a headache now and can eat cheese, providing she has only one egg a fortnight. She says she can eat cakes or anything made with eggs in the cooking.

Jennifer who discovered she was allergic to poultry and eggs some years ago can now eat poultry once a week and small quantities of egg without problems. However she must keep off omelettes, which she finds very difficult as she really misses them. She says: 'Twice I have been overcome by temptation but never again. It really was not worth it. A few minutes of mouth watering pleasure gives hours and hours of displeasure.'

## Testing a food

How do you test whether a food, drink or ingredient really is the cause of your allergy? The easiest way is to eat it and see, or more accurately, feel the result. Start by eating only a small amount as you may possibly get a strong reaction. If you start reacting, stop eating that food. If you do not get any symptoms, continue, gradually increasing the amount you eat each time. But if your allergy returns, remember that that food may be the cause. Eliminate it and see.

There is a view that if you do not eat a food to which you are allergic for some time, perhaps six months or a year, you lose your vulnerability to it. This is something you may care to test at some stage. However many people are unwilling to do this for fear of making themselves ill again. Why inflict symptoms on yourself or your child unnecessarily?

However accidents do happen and this is when most people have been able to prove their point. When eating out in someone else's home for instance, you may be reluctant to refuse a dish offered. This may contain the suspect food and yet you eat it to please your host. If you are ill afterwards, you will realise the cause.

An adult can find ways of refusing food politely. But a child may find this more difficult. Often he does not want to be different from other children and he may accept the forbidden food, especially if he is encouraged to do so.

Margaret's son is such an example. This is her story: 'I am blessed with a young son who verges on the hyperactive. Very early on our doctor advised that he never be given tea, coffee or cola drink, all high in caffeine. It has been difficult to police as he is a very gregarious child and there have been occasional lapses when he has spent a few hours in the homes of new friends and I have forgotten to warn the mums.' Chocolate also contains caffeine.

'At four and a half he is reasonably good and usually says, "I am not allowed that" when offered; but some people have been known to say things like "Oh, go on, I won't tell your Mum" as if they thought he was being deprived. And, of course, he gives in to temptation just like the rest of us. On these occasions he has been heavily over-active, noisy and often almost uncontrollably wild in

his movements, shrieking, yelling and rushing around quite
pointlessly.'

## Addiction or aversion?

From my own research there seems little guide between adoring a
food which causes an allergy and hating it, although some experts
have said that a craving for a food may be an indication. Dr Theron
Randolph, a specialist in allergy in America, believes you may be
addicted to a food like an alcoholic is addicted to drink.[8]

Here are two examples I received which show both sides of the
coin: one of a little girl who was allergic to the milk she loved; the
other of a young boy who wisely, if unknowingly, refused the eggs
and nuts which made him ill.

Sue's four year old daughter developed very bad sleeping habits
from the age of 16 months due to milk which the child loved. This
gradually got worse until she was only sleeping four hours a night.
Sue says: 'In desperation I went to my doctor who said it could be
an allergy to something, especially as her behaviour during the day
was getting worse – temper tantrums which were really bad,
fidgeting, she could not even sit still long enough to eat a meal. She
would spend a lot of time running round in circles. She also became
very aggressive, especially towards me. Under guidance from my
doctor I kept her off certain foods – colouring, preservatives etc.
Nothing made any difference so eventually he said to try avoiding
cows' milk. She loved milk and anything to do with it – yogurt,
cheese etc. After keeping her off it for 24 hours she slept for 12
hours. Amazing but it worked. After only a couple of weeks her
behaviour improved as well.'

Ruth's son, on the other hand, cannot eat eggs or nuts including
peanuts (although they are not part of the nut family). She says:
'We discovered his allergy to egg white when he was one year old.
My health visitor had warned me he might be allergic to egg
because he refused to eat eggs at all. However I forgot about this so
I made his first birthday cake with Royal Icing made with a raw egg
white. After eating some, he had a violent reaction.'

The reaction of Ruth's son was to swell up all over and vomit.
The swelling was very itchy. He also gets this reaction if he eats nuts

(except coconut). Ruth adds: 'He could never bear the smell of nuts or peanut butter and after accidentally eating a chocolate containing nuts and being quite ill, we realised he was also allergic to nuts. In fact, he is so allergic to nuts, he cannot touch anyone who has just eaten them. I once had a peanut butter sandwich and then gave him a cuddle. Where I had kissed him on his face he became itchy and swollen.'

Do not force yourself to eat a food you do not like. Similarly do not force your child to eat a food to which he or she seems to have taken a dislike. If you feel you are addicted to a particular food or drink and think it might be a cause of your allergy, cut it out. If you are addicted, you may suffer some withdrawal symptoms but these usually last only a couple of days.

## How to treat your child

It is very important that you do not make your child feel a freak or that he is at fault because of his allergy. Speak to him openly and frankly about the allergy and foods which you feel may be causing his symptoms. Obviously your child will feel different from other children as they can eat things he cannot but no child likes to be ill so if you explain that certain foods or drink may be causing this, he will probably agree only too readily to avoid them.

It will depend on your child's age how deeply you discuss with him what foods or drink are causing his allergy. But if you talk comfortably and factually about the connection, he will be more willing to co-operate and may well come up with some ideas of his own. Also he may suggest a food which could have caused a current attack or admit that he did, in fact, eat a 'forbidden' one.

If you discover he has eaten a 'bad' food and he denies it, do not press the point. Just state that if he did eat that food, this may be why he is now suffering. If he did really eat it, he will know and be aware of the relationship; and will probably remember it the next time he is tempted.

Always try to treat your child normally. Do not fuss over him or seem overconcerned. Difficult advice I know. But children get anxious if they see you worry about them. And that can do not good at all. Also do not treat your child too softly. If he has been naughty, do not be afraid to scold him. A child who feels he can get away with murder whilst wheezing badly or nursing a headache for instance, will use it as a weapon against you in the future.

## Non-food causes of allergies

Not all allergies are caused by food or drink. Many people suffer from hayfever caused by grass or other pollens whilst others sneeze or react in different ways when near an animal, a cat for example. Some people react to gas or petrol fumes in the environment. Listed below are the more common irritants to consider alongside your investigation into food.

## In the home

**House dust and house dust mites,** tiny creatures which live in house dust, can cause allergies, especially asthma and hayfever and to a lesser degree, eczema and urticaria (hives).

If your symptoms get worse whilst dusting or cleaning, house dust may be a cause. A friend of mine is a nurse who visits patients at home. She says that if the blankets on the bed are dusty, she immediately gets an itchy nose and throat and tight chest.

House dust mites measure less than ½ mm. and usually live in bedding, mattresses and carpets and thrive in damp homes with poor ventilation. They may also live in heavy winter clothes which are not often washed. It is their faeces (droppings) which cause allergy.

Skin testing can show if you are allergic to house dust mites but occasionally it may show a skin reaction in people who do not suffer from that irritant.

Unfortunately it is almost impossible to eliminate house dust mites from the home although regularly airing beds and vacuum cleaning carpets may help a bit. It means living in an almost bare house with no carpets, rugs or curtains and all surfaces must be smooth and cleaned regularly (at least once a day) so no dust particles can settle. Even under laboratory conditions, it was found impossible to eliminate more than 70 per cent of house dust mites and in two days half of the original number had returned. When a group of mothers tried to eradicate house dust mites from their children's beds under clinical supervision, the results were shown to be ineffective.[9] Keeping a bedroom cool (68°F or lower) may reduce the amount of dust in the air.[10]

**Feather pillows and furniture stuffing.** If your allergy occurs only at night, it may be your feather pillow or down quilt causing it. If you suddenly get worse sitting in a particular chair or near it, suspect that chair. Upholstered furniture and beds may be stuffed with horse hair or other fibres which can cause allergy. Foam rubber stuffing may also cause trouble for some people.

**Household goods and chemicals.** Cleaning materials, like polish, oven cleaner or powerful disinfectants, may give off fumes which affect you. Air fresheners and other perfumed sprays and aerosols, including insect sprays, may also cause reactions because they leave tiny droplets in the air which are inhaled. Washing-up liquid can act in the same way – to avoid this, squeeze the container with its nozzle under water. Dishes should be rinsed thoroughly.

**Gas fumes.** If you think fumes from your gas stove, heater or boiler are causing your allergy, you may have to consider replacing them with an electric equivalent. Make sure there are no gas leaks, e.g. a pilot light blown out. Gas appliances use up oxygen in the room when they burn which may make an asthma sufferer have an attack or get worse merely because of the reduction of oxygen in the air. Headaches and other symptoms may also get worse. This may occur more in winter when windows and doors are tightly shut.

**Cooking fumes,** e.g. fried foods, may cause symptoms.

**Plastic and rubber.** When the weather is hot, or if your home is kept at a very warm temperature, plastic and rubber may give off fumes and cause a reaction. The softer the plastic, the more likely it is to give off fumes. Watch out for balloons and laminated (shiny) book covers. Also rubber pillows and mattresses or plastic-covered mattresses and plastic curtains. Plastic containers may affect the food they hold.

**Paint and varnish**. When your home is being painted or wood varnished, the fumes may have an adverse affect on you. Most paints nowadays are plastic based.

**Pens, pencils and children's paints**. Don't suck, or let your child suck, the tops of pens and pencils and stop, if you can, a child with paint on his hands putting them in his mouth. Dust from chalk may also affect some people.

**Glue**, either heavy duty or the sort your child may use, can give off fumes. Similarly don't lick stamps or envelopes if you think they may affect you. Use a small damp sponge.

**Tobacco smoke** is harmful to smokers and may affect other people standing nearby. If someone is bothered by tobacco smoke, do not smoke in the same room or in a closed car. Best of all, give up the habit.

**Animals** can cause allergic symptoms, usually asthma, hayfever, eczema or other rashes. Cats seem to be the most common cause. Horses come next. Some people may have an allergic reaction even if the animal is not in the room. I received one letter from a lady who visited a friend and after a disturbed night was told that a pet cat usually slept on her bed. A circus owner told my husband that, when a group of asthmatic children visited her circus, even when seated right at the back, many would start coughing and wheezing when the animals entered the ring.

## What you wear

**Fabrics** including wool and fur may bring out an allergic reaction in some people. One lady thought she was allergic to her husband until she discovered it was his tweed jacket which was causing the trouble.

**Washing powders and fabric softeners** can cause skin conditions if the washed clothes are worn next to the skin. Biological washing powders (which contain special enzymes) are particularly suspect.

Rashes on babies' bottoms may be caused by nappies washed in these powders. Washing powders also contain perfume and whiteners which may cause trouble. Inhaling the dust from washing powders (especially those for automatic dishwashers) or even standing over the sink using them may cause a reaction in some people.

**Dry cleaned clothes** may give off troublesome vapours.

**Perfumed and coloured toiletries** such as soap, cleansing and moisturising creams, shampoo, talc and hairspray may cause irritation. Silvia found that spraying her neck with perfume produced a rash but says she gets no reaction if she applies perfume 'carefully with my finger behind the ears in the old-fashioned way.'

**Make-up.** Silvia also found she could not use any green eye make-up as it made her eyes swell: 'like a frog's, discoloured and lined, a very depressing experience'. She says she cannot eat any food with green colouring in it either. Other cosmetics as well as nail polish and remover may cause trouble to some people.

## Out of doors

**Pollen.** Trees, plants and grasses pollinate at different times of the year and any of these pollens may affect you. One in ten people in the UK are believed to suffer hayfever from grass pollen. Common grasses pollinate from the middle of May to the end of August but if the weather has been warm and wet during April and May, the season may start earlier and possibly be more severe. The season starts up to four weeks later in the north of Britain than in the south. The first trees to pollinate are the alder and hazel in the middle of February or March but the chief troublemakers in the UK are thought to be the silver birch in April and the plane in May. Trees vary in the time taken to pollinate but they are at their worst for one to three weeks.

Trees and plants pollinate in different ways. Those which blossom beautifully every year are unlikely to cause your allergy as they use bees and other insects to carry their pollen for them.

Grass, on the other hand, and trees which do not have noticeable flowers, need the wind, and favourable weather conditions, to scatter their pollen. Such pollen is very light, invisible to the naked eye, and can be blown for up to 30 miles on dry, warm and windy days but if it rains appreciably, the pollen grains, together with other dusts, become damp, fall to the ground and should not bother you. Pollen can trouble you during the evening and night as well as during the day although often the highest level is reported during the late afternoon. Keep windows shut, if possible, and air your home early in the morning. The best place to escape pollen is at the seaside where a sea breeze will blow any pollen away from you.

During June and July the Asthma Research Council publishes the grass pollen count for London during the previous 24 hours. This together with a forecast of what the count is likely to be can be heard by ringing the Telephone Weather Forecast (01-246 8091). Over 50 grains is considered high and likely to affect anyone suffering from hayfever. Currently there is no national service providing a pollen count for the rest of the country.

If you keep your diaries for over a year, you may notice that a tree or plant flowers or buds at almost exactly the same time every year. This may indicate the time of year you start to react; yet it may not be that particular plant or tree which causes the trouble but something else pollinating at the same time (usually within a few days) each year.

**Mould spores.** Moulds are part of the fungus family. Some grow in the fields and countryside but others may be found in any damp place including basements, badly aired rooms and under kitchen sinks and baths where water can seep through. The moulds throw off spores into the air which are very light and can be blown long distances. These spores, like pollen, are inhaled through your nose and mouth and then into your lungs and can cause hayfever and asthma. Some mould spores are at their worst during late summer and autumn but others fly around from spring to autumn, especially in warm damp conditions. A research project in New Zealand showed that even during the pollen season, there were more mould spores in the air than pollen.[9]

**Exhaust fumes** from cars and lorries are difficult to avoid unless you live in the heart of the country but here are a few hints. Avoid walking along main roads during rush-hours. Avoid crossing roads with children in pushchairs when cars have stopped in front of you: the child will get a full blast of fumes from the exhaust pipe. If you are travelling in a car, wind up the windows in heavy or low moving traffic and while going through tunnels.

**Swimming pools.** Disinfectants, including chlorine, and fungicides are added to the water of swimming pools. These may cause eye, skin or other complaints to sensitive swimmers. There is also a high concentration of moulds around swimming pools.

# Clinical testing for allergies

There are several ways of testing for allergies which may help you discover the cause of yours. But unfortunately for everyone who thinks they may help, there are others who do not.

**Skin testing** is carried out within the National Health Service. The skin is either scratched with the substance thought to be causing the allergy or the substance is injected under the skin. Although thought to be 80 per cent accurate in detecting allergy to pollen in hayfever sufferers, it is not thought to be effective in discovering food causes.[11]

**Blood testing** is also carried out under the National Health Service in some hospitals. Again there is divided opinion as to how useful this is in helping the patient discover any food allergy.

**Hair testing.** Although thought by many doctors and shown by some reports in the press to be unreliable, some people have found hair testing helpful. Jennifer discovered her allergy to poultry and eggs through having her hair tested. She said her hair had to be absolutely clean, washed with a natural shampoo from a health shop and left to dry naturally. About 20 hairs were then cut from the crown of her head and analysed. She was most sceptical of the outcome but after avoiding the offending foods, she felt much better and became worse if she ate them again.

**Pulse testing** is also thought to be unreliable. But Margaret says she discovered milk was causing her asthma by this method. She was told by her doctor to take her pulse before eating certain foods and then 20 minutes and an hour afterwards. On drinking milk her pulse rate increased quite remarkably.

**Notes**

1  A set of 12 *Allergy? Think About Food* charts, price £1·95 plus 40p p&p, is available from Wisebuy Publications, PO Box 379, London NW3 1NJ.

2  *Is Migraine Food Allergy?*, J. Egger et al, The Lancet, 15 October 1983.

3  *Food Intolerance and Food Aversion*, a joint report of the Royal College of Physicians and the British Nutrition Foundation, April 1984.

4  *False food allergies: non-specific reactions to foodstuffs*, D.A. Moneret-Vautrin; *Migraine*, Edda Hanington, published in *Clinical Reactions to Food* edited by M.H. Lessof, John Wiley & Sons 1983.

5  *Medicines, A Guide for Everybody*, Peter Parish, Penguin Reference Books, 1982, p.297.

6  *Why Your Child is Hyperactive*, Ben. F. Feingold, Random House, New York, 1975.

7  *Controlled trial of oligoantigenic treatment in the hyperkinetic syndrome*, J. Egger et al, the Lancet, 9 March 1985.

8  *An Alternative Approach to Allergies*, Theron G. Randolph and Ralph W. Moss, Bantam Books, 1980. Published in the UK by Thorsons.

9  Information supplied by the Asthma Research Council.

10  *Chemical Victims*, Dr Richard Mackarness, Pan, 1980.

11  Dr Keith Eaton in his talk to the Society of Environmental Therapy Conference, London, March 1984.

12  *Salicylates, oligoantigenic diets, and behaviour*, Anne Swain et al, The Lancet, 6 July 1985.

13  *Salicylates in foods*, Anne R. Swain et al, Journal of the American Dietetic Association, August 1985.

# 4

# Labelling

When you are researching into which food or foods may be causing
your allergy, carefully study the labels, in particular the list of
ingredients, on all the processed food you buy. Your shopping may
take longer at first but it is essential if you want to assess whether a
particular food or ingredient is really causing the trouble.

Do not judge the product simply by the name on its container.
Manufacturers put different ingredients into very similar sounding
and looking products so it is not sufficient to think that one bottle
of mayonnaise is the same as another or all gravy mixes contain the
same ingredients. You will have to read each individual list. Even
crisps with exactly the same flavour produced by the same
manufacturer have been known to contain different additives if
their shapes are different.

Some products may mislead the consumer into thinking they are
additive free. They advertise 'no preservatives' in prominent
lettering even if they contain colouring; alternatively they announce
'no colouring' but contain other additives. Beefburgers
proclaiming they are 100 per cent beef may contain additives as
well. The list of ingredients is your most accurate guide although it
may not give you all the information you need.

This chapter relates to the latest Food Labelling Regulations
brought into effect on 1 July 1986. It tells you how the law stands at
the moment with regard to what information must be disclosed.

## Foods not requiring full labelling

Broadly speaking unpacked foods like bacon, cooked meat and bread, and food packed by the shopkeeper need not be labelled with their ingredients but must be marked or labelled with an indication of certain additives – antioxidants, artificial sweeteners, colours, flavour enhancers, flavourings or preservatives. Unpacked or see-through packed flour confectionery such as cakes, shortbread, crumpets, macaroons and pastry, and ice-cream need not be so marked provided there is a notice nearby stating that these types of additives may have been used. Watch out for these unlabelled foods as they may contain many ingredients you wish to avoid, both natural like wheat and eggs or artifical such as colouring and preservatives. Unless you can ask and be sure of the ingredients, you may find it safer to buy the packaged, labelled version.

Both unpacked and packed foods sold at a delicatessen counter should also state either on a label or on a notice nearby if they contain any of the additives mentioned in the previous paragraph. However this rule seems to be ignored, possibly legally, in some delicatessen shops which may claim to be take-away restaurants. Take-away and sit-down restaurants need only name their merchandise; whether the food is hot or cold, packed on the premises or unpacked, the ingredients need not be disclosed. Watch out for food like salami, bacon, cheese and mixed salads which may contain undisclosed ingredients.

**Small packages of food** (less than 10 square centimetres of the largest surface) need only be marked with the name of the food and a datemark (if required by law). This is despite a recommendation made by the Food Standards Committee[1] that ingredients should be declared even on small containers.

**Chocolate and cocoa products**, including those coming in bars, wrappers and boxes, need only list certain details of their contents, for example, the minimum percentage of cocoa and milk solids. The use of additives, including colours and preservatives, need not be disclosed. A couple of manufacturers are naming them but unfortunately the majority are not. The Food Standards Committee said: 'A full list of ingredients would provide more useful information to consumers than a partial declaration and we see no reason why all the ingredients should not be named'.

The lack of information is shown in this example of some Swiss chocolate sold in this country. The part of the label displaying the contents in Swiss (French and German) was covered by the English declaration of: 'Milk chocolate contains Cocoa Solids 35%, Milk Solids 14% min.' In French and German the following ingredients were listed: sugar, nuts, cocoa butter, cocoa solids, almonds, milk powder, vegetable fat, skimmed milk powder, wafer biscuit, sorbitol, emulsifier (lecithin), modified starch, flavouring, colourings.

**Other prepacked foods** which do not have to list their ingredients are fresh fruit and vegetables which have not been peeled or cut into pieces; carbonated water to which only carbon dioxide has been added; vinegar, sugar, honey, dried and condensed milk each made from a single product and any other food consisting of one ingredient; cheese, butter, fermented milk and fermented cream containing only lactic products, enzymes, micro-organism cultures and salt in the case of cheese (except curd and processed cheese); and flavourings themselves.

**Home-made** food sold for charity does not have to be labelled. And food and drink supplied under Government contract to British or visiting armed forces do not come under the Regulations at all.

## Labelled foods

Apart from those mentioned above, prepacked food and drink must be labelled with the following details:
• The name of the food.
• A list of ingredients.
• The net weight or volume.
• A datemark.
• Any special storage instructions.
• Instructions on how to use the product if necessary.

• The name and address of the manufacturer, packer or seller within the European Community (Common Market); and sometimes the place or country where the food comes from.

Labels should be easy to read and understand with all words visible and not hidden by other labels fixed on top. As you will learn when you become a regular label reader, this is not always the case. Ingredients are often difficult to find on the label or packet perhaps printed sideways or in very small type, or the price label is stuck right over the sell by date or list of ingredients.

## The name of the food

Food and drink should be accurately named. 'The name of the food must not mislead the customer' says a leaflet issued by the Ministry of Agriculture entitled 'Look At The Label' which explains the labelling regulations. The leaflet gives the following example: 'Strawberry yogurt for instance can only be called "strawberry" or "strawberry flavoured" yogurt, or have a picture of strawberries on the label, if its flavour comes mainly from real strawberries. If it tastes of strawberries, but the flavour is not mainly from the fruit, it can be called "strawberry flavour" yogurt'.

You may have to read this example a couple of times to discover that 'flavour' and 'flavoured' can mean two very different things.

The Food Standards Committee felt these descriptions were not sufficiently clear. They said: 'A much more positive distinction needs to be drawn on labels between the use of artificial flavour and the use of the "real" food as the source of the flavour. In our view this will only be achieved by the use of the term "artificial flavour" which without any shadow of doubt indicates that the flavour has not been derived from a "natural" source in the sense understood by the public.'

They then went on to recommend that, where a food is described as 'X flavour', the words 'contains artificial flavour' should appear on the label nearby and be printed in the same size, style and colour. They defined 'artificial flavour' as any flavouring substance which was not derived exclusively from the fruit named. Unfortunately their recommendation was ignored.

## List of ingredients

Ingredients must be listed in order of their weight, the heaviest ingredient at the top of the list, the lightest at the bottom. The amount used need not be revealed although the Food Standards Committee expressed the view that percentage declarations, especially of the main ingredient, of certain foods and drinks would be useful to the public.

Some ingredients need not be fully identified. For instance fats and oils need only be described as vegetable or animal, the particular vegetable or animal they are made from can remain anonymous. Cheese, fish, meat, nuts, herbs, spices and starch can also be described in these terms: the type of cheese, fish etc. need not necessarily be named.

Water added as an ingredient must be declared if it makes up more than 5 per cent of the weight of the finished product. But it is not named in the case of fruit juices which are reconstituted from concentrate (see p.100) or other foods which have had their water content withdrawn and then replaced with other water.

The use of the following categories of food additives must be listed: acids, acidity regulators, anti-caking agents, anti-foaming agents, antioxidants, artificial sweeteners, colours, emulsifiers, emulsifying salts, flavour enhancers, flavours, flour improvers, gelling agents, glazing agents, preservatives, raising agents, stabilisers and thickeners.

Apart from flavourings, all these additives must be indentified by their category name eg colour, preservative, flavour enhancer, and be followed by either their individual chemical name or more usually their code number. For instance the food colouring tartrazine will usually appears as 'Colour: E102'. A full list of these additives and their code numbers is given in Appendix 2.

Occasionally whilst shopping after 1 July 1986 you may still find processed foods which do not give full details. They might just say colour but not say which one. This is allowable by law if the product was actually manufactured before 1 January 1986. If you are concerned, either do not buy the product or ring the manufacturer to enquire which additive it is.

## Ingredients of ingredients

Some foods contain ingredients which are themselves made of two or more ingredients, for instance biscuits may contain margarine which is made of vegetable oil, salt, emulsifiers, colouring, flavouring and usually whey. The names of these ingredients of ingredients should normally be disclosed; either by stating the combined ingredient and then listing its ingredients, e.g. margarine (vegetable oil, salt, emulsifiers etc.); or by listing only the individual ingredients without reference to the name of the combined ingredient e.g. vegetable oil, salt etc. and no mention of margarine.

The exceptions to this rule are when the ingredients of the combined ingredient would not normally be disclosed if it was sold on its own e.g. chocolate; or if the combined ingredient constitutes less than 25 per cent of the finished product e.g. mustard in a frozen meat dish, but if that combined ingredient contains an additive, the category of additive should be named, e.g. salami contains preservative so a pizza containing salami should disclose preservative on the label.

Unfortunately there are some loopholes in the law. For instance the Food Labelling Regulations state that an additive need not be named if 'its presence is due solely to the fact it was contained in an ingredient of the food, if it serves no significant technological function in the finished product'. This means, for example, that a preservative used in fruit which is later made into jam, but which is not enough to preserve the jam, does not need to be declared on the jam label. It also means that an antioxidant used in vegetable oil which is then used to fry crisps need not be declared on a packet of crisps if the antioxidant was only there to preserve the oil and not the crisps.

Another loop-hole is when 'an additive is used solely as a processing aid'. This explains why bleaching agents in white flour need not be disclosed. Also 'any substance other than water which is used as a solvent or carrier for an additive and is used in an amount that is no more than that which is strictly necessary for that purpose' need not be disclosed.

Because of the complexity of these regulations, you should be extremely careful about eating anything which contains an ingredient which itself might contain an additive although none is mentioned on the label. At the time of going to press, I am still seeing margarine and salami as an ingredient on packets and the fact that they contain additives is not always disclosed.

Additives put into animal feed to make egg yolks yellower and trout and salmon pinker will never be revealed. Nor will colouring injected in to orange tree trunks to make the fruit a better colour.[2] Read about these individual foods later in the book. Animal feed may contain any colouring which is allowed in food if the feed is made of human waste, e.g. broken biscuits.

## Read and keep your labels

Read labels carefully before you buy prepared foods if you wish to avoid certain additives or ingredients. If you are unsure about the content of a particular food, for instance you need to know what kind of vegetable or animal fat is used, phone or write to the name and address on the label. The Quality Controller or Public Relations Officer is usually the man or woman to ask for. On the whole I have found that manufacturers are very helpful especially if you explain why you are anxious to know more. So do not be afraid to ask.

Keep labels for a while. Write on them the date you bought them. You may need to refer to them if you suddenly discover you or your child might be allergic to something you had not previously suspected. Your diary may only note that you had, for instance, a particular brand of soup or frozen food. This way you can check up on what exactly has been eaten in the past. Store labels in a small box in the kitchen. This should not take up much space and will be convenient for you to use.

## Inaccurate labelling

Occasionally errors or omissions occur on labels and all the ingredients or additives are not declared. I came across this example in November 1984. While looking through the freezer cabinet of my local supermarket I noticed that a packet of Blue Crest Golden Breaded Haddock Fillets looked very orange but declared no colouring. Next to that packet was one containing Golden Breaded Cod Fillets produced by the same manufacturer. This package declared on its label the colours E102 (tartrazine) and E110 (sunset yellow) plus the flavour enhancer monosodium glutamate (621). After investigation it was revealed that the haddock fillets also contained these additives. Blue Crest subsequently amended its labelling.

Although difficult to discover such omissions, if you do suspect the possibility, ask the manufacturer listed on the label. Alternatively contact the Trading Standards Officer at your local town hall who can analyse the product and discover the truth. In Scotland or London, the person to approach is the Environmental Health Officer also at your local town hall.

**Notes**

1 The Food Standards Committee was a group of professors, chemists, lawyers, manufacturing and consumer representatives appointed by the Ministry of Agriculture, Fisheries and Food to recommend revisions to the food regulations. Their report on Food Labelling was published in 1975. This committee has now been replaced by the similarly constituted Food Advisory Committee.

2 Reported in *Food Additives*, Erik Millstone, Penguin Special, 1986.

# 5

# Everyday foods

The foods described in this chapter are those you eat most days: fish, fruit, meat, nuts and vegetables. They make up the bulk of your diet – alongside wheat and dairy products which are described in the next two chapters.

Buy these foods in their natural state: uncooked and unprocessed. Canned or bottled foods usually contain other ingredients or additives; frozen foods may do. Why you should avoid most of the additives mentioned in the next five chapters is explained in Chapter 10. While searching for individual foods which may cause you trouble, you will find it much more difficult if you are eating too many mixtures. Simplify your food as far as possible.

I have given examples from the letters I received to show that a particular food can cause an allergy. Do not assume that you must be allergic to the same food just because the symptoms described appear remarkably like your own. These examples are here to show what can happen, not what must happen. They are just given as a guide. If you automatically think 'My goodness, I can't eat that . . . and that . . . and that', you will make your life pretty miserable and unnecessarily so.

Go by your diary and chart to see if any of these foods are consistently eaten before an attack but check whether they have been eaten and you have been perfectly all right afterwards (for the next 24 hours or so). Do not jump too readily to conclusions. Your diary will help you see reason.

## Fish

There are many varieties of fish: cod, plaice, haddock, salmon, mackerel and herring to name but a few. Each one should be considered individually. Shellfish, associated with allergies for many centuries, should also be thought of individually. My mother is extremely sick whenever she eats prawns and has found scampi affect her in the same way. However she can eat crab.

The following three examples show that some people can tolerate certain fish but not others. Joan found she developed a constricted throat, swollen lips and itching eyes whenever she ate plaice, salmon, trout and shellfish but she says cod, halibut, kippers and sardines do her no harm. She freely admits that she does not know why. A lady from Newcastle mentions that only shellfish make her get eczema on her face and neck. By contrast a letter from Cheshire reveals that three members of the family, mother, son and daughter, can eat shellfish (crab, prawns and shrimps) but not white fish like cod.

According to Erik Millstone[5] salmon and trout which are reared on fish farms may be given food containing red colouring to make their flesh pinker. This will not be disclosed. The colouring used is canthaxanthin (E161g).

**Smoked fish,** whether bought over the fresh fish counter or prepacked, must be regarded with suspicion. Smoked cod and haddock are likely to be coloured yellow with tartrazine (E102) or sunset yellow (E110) and kippers with brown FK (E154). Smoked salmon and mackerel may also be coloured as well as having salt and sugar added. You will find it safer to buy smoked fish which is prepacked and labelled rather than from your fishmonger who may not reveal any colouring used. There is also the possibility of an allergy to the smoke itself.

**Frozen fish** with nothing added to it is a good way of buying fish if you cannot buy fresh. Ice glaze, sometimes called protective glaze, is mentioned on some packets. It consists of plain water which may have been chlorinated. The glaze is used to protect fish from drying out.

**Frozen battered or breadcrumbed fish and fishfingers** are coated with bread or flour (made from wheat) and oil, the source of which will not be identified. The batter or breadcrumbs may contain yellow colouring, often tartrazine (E102), to make the covering look golden and other additives such as monosodium glutamate (621) may be used. If you suspect any of the ingredients on the label, avoid the product.

**Frozen fish dinners** with sauces contain many ingredients and additives. Check the list of ingredients carefully.

**Canned fish.** Canned tuna and salmon are two of the few canned products I buy as there is usually nothing added except salt or vegetable oil (the vegetable is never named). Mackerel and anchovies also come under this category. Canned fish with other ingredients, e.g. tomatoes, tend not to contain preservatives or other additives to the same extent as, say, canned meat products: but always check the labels to see if any of the ingredients are likely to disagree with you. High levels of histamine (see p.76) may accumulate in canned fish kept a long time. Unfortunately canned fish does not have to be date marked.

**Fish spread and paste** are made from many substances. Look at the label carefully before buying.

**How to help yourself with fish.** Consider each type of fish separately.
 • Look out for it as an ingredient in other foods.
 • The amount of histamine in canned fish increases the longer the tin is kept. Although there is no way of knowing how long a can of fish has been kept in a shop, avoid buying in bulk and leaving the cans in your storecupboard for many months.
 • Fish and shellfish are thought by some doctors to have a histamine-releasing action (see p.76).
 • Remember to check the ingredients and additives on the labels of smoked, frozen and canned fish; it may be an added ingredient which is causing your allergy.

# Fruit

Oranges and other citrus fruit, strawberries, apples, grapes and bananas were all mentioned more than once by the people who wrote to me about their allergies. The allergies they attributed to fruit are shown in Appendix 3. Fruits containing salicylate (see p.76) were also avoided by some people. Rhubarb, plums, pears, pineapple and blackcurrants were only mentioned once.

Eczema sufferers seem worst affected by fruit: oranges were quoted by five people and strawberries by four. Diane wrote about her seven year old son who suffers from eczema: 'I have been unable to pinpont any particular food which makes my son's eczema react except apples, which immediately bring him out in a rash and also anything containing blackcurrant.'

Fruit is generally good for you so do not eliminate any fruit from your diet permanently unless you have proved to yourself that it is causing your allergy.

**Oranges, satsumas, tangerines and clementines** may contain colouring which is injected into the fruit tree. This will not be disclosed.[5]

**Fruit juice,** made from a fruit and containing nothing else, should be considered in the same way as the fruit itself. There is usually nothing added to fruit juice though it may contain the skin and pulp as well as the juice; the only other ingredient allowed is sugar which must be disclosed on the label. Most fruit juice is 'made from concentrate' which means that water is taken out of the fruit in the country of origin and put back (sometimes from the tap) when it is packed into its carton, bottle or tin. If you are allergic to tap water, you may react to this sort of fruit juice: buy the concentrate, usually frozen, instead and dilute it yourself with bottled water. Do not confuse fruit juice with squash or other drinks which contain many ingredients and additives besides the fruit (see p.149).

**Dried fruit.** Often contains preservatives, usually sulphur dioxide (E220). Check on the label before buying.

**Canned fruit** often contains only the fruit and perhaps some sugar. Study labels carefully to ensure colouring and preservatives have not been added.

**How to help yourself with fruit.** Consider each fruit separately although if you are allergic to oranges you may also be allergic to other citrus fruits like grapefruit, lemons, limes, tangerines, clementines and satsumas.

• If you are allergic to citrus fruit, you may possibly be affected by citric acid (E330) and its derivatives: E331, E332, E333, 380, 381 and E472(c) although these additives are usually prepared from malasses (sugar). Pectin (E440), used as a gelling agent in jams and jellies, may be made from the peel of citrus fruit.

• Wash all fruit carefully.

• If you find you react to most fruit, your allergy may be caused by the chemical fungicides and pesticides which are regularly sprayed onto most fruit. A survey in 1983 carried out by the Association of Public Analysts showed that almost a third of fruit sold in high street shops was found to have detectable levels of pesticide residues. Washing the fruit will not get rid of the contaminants completely and it may help to peel the fruit. Only do this if you feel convinced that spraying is the cause of your allergy as most of the vitamins and minerals lie just beneath the skin. Buying organically grown fruit may be an alternative[4] or grow your own if you have the space.

• Some imported apples, usually North American, are coated in wax to give them a shinier appearance. English apples are not waxed.

• Check for additives in canned and dried fruit.

• Do not mistake fruit juice for squash or other drinks. It is not juice unless it is described as juice on the label. Check for added ingredients. If none are stated on the carton or bottle, you can assume there are none.

• Strawberries, pineapple and pawpaw are thought to have a histamine-releasing action (see p.76).

• Many fruits contain salicylate (see p. 76).

## Meat

Think of meat as beef, pork, lamb and chicken, not simply as meat. Only one letter said that all meats were the cause of allergy; they gave a little boy eczema. Five people felt beef was a cause; three said it caused eczema, one said it was responsible for cold-like symptoms causing temporary deafness. These four also eliminated milk from their diet. One said it caused wheezing.

Four people quoted chicken as one of the causes of cold-like symptoms (the person who could not each beef), eczema, stomach complaint (similar to mild food poisoning) and depression. Two of these also cut out eggs. Lamb was reported twice, once causing eczema and once migraine. Pork was also named twice: once as causing catarrh, and once as causing migraine (to the same lady who could not eat lamb).

**Is meat good for you?** There is a popular view that the western world eats too much meat and adults should cut down their consumption of it. This is because animal fat is believed to contribute to heart disease and strokes. However Dr Richard Mackarness puts forward an alternative view. He believes that man is meant to eat meat and his 'caveman' diet is based on this assumption. He feels that meat has been substituted by too much grain (wheat, corn etc.) and other processed, over-refined foods and recommends lamb as a meat which causes very little allergic reaction.[1]

If your child suffers from allergy but can eat meat, or certain types of meat, do not cut down on the quantity he or she eats. Children need the protein, vitamins and minerals it contains.

**Sausages, salami, paté, spread and fresh meat pies** contain many ingredients and additives other than meat. These should be labelled on the packet: check through the ingredients and if you suspect anything, do not buy it. Avoid buying these items over the deli-counter unless there is a label on the wrapping telling you what they contain. Don't just go by a notice nearby. I have found they can be inaccurate. Although they should state all additives used, I recently saw a marker above a salami on sale at a butchers shop stating that it contained preservative. On examining the label on the wrapping, I discovered the salami contained other additives including the flavour enhancer monosodium glutamate (621). Try making your own sausages with some finely minced lamb or beef and add some herbs and seasoning which you know you can tolerate. Sausages do not need a 'skin' to stay intact.

**Ready-prepared chilled meat portions.** You will often see chicken, and perhaps other meats, already cooked and flavoured in the chilling chests of many supermarkets. Check the ingredients before you buy. Often printed in very small lettering, they may reveal additives, e.g. colouring, you can well do without.

**Frozen meat.** If meat has been frozen and is then sold thawed, this must be declared on the label with the words 'previously frozen – do not refreeze'. If the meat is not prepacked, these words must be on a notice nearby.

**Frozen hamburgers and other meat products.** You can now buy many frozen meals which have meat as their main ingredient but which contain other ingredients and additives as well. Frozen hamburgers are the most popular example. Most frozen meat products contain the additives: flavour enhancer, preservative and colouring. Avoid these if you can and make your own. For instance, home-made hamburgers with fresh minced beef or lamb and a little salt or pepper added (plus a little chopped onion if you like) are just as delicious and contain no artificial additives or thickeners.

**Canned meat products** contain many ingredients. Each one must be thought about individually. For instance it may not be the meat which is the cause of the trouble, it may be the tomato or other vegetable, it may be a milk product like caseinate (milk protein) or cheese, or modified starch (which is made from wheat or corn). It could also be the many additives like colouring, preservatives or flavour enhancer which go into the making of these products. All cans disclose on their labels the ingredients and additives which have gone into the making of the product; it is up to you to check through them.

**How to help yourself with meat.** Try and identify which type of meat you are allergic to, e.g. beef, lamb, pork, chicken, duck.

• Eat fresh meat rather than frozen or canned. It may be more expensive but is worth the extra money if your or your child's health is at stake.

• Grill and roast; avoid frying if possible.

• Suet is animal fat, often beef fat.

• Gelatine is made from beef bones.

• Veal is young beef.

• If you are allergic to beef, you may also be allergic to milk and other dairy products.

• If you are allergic to pork, you will also be allergic to bacon, ham and lard.

• Cured and smoked meat, e.g. bacon and ham, may contain salt, sodium nitrite (E250) and possibly sodium or potassium nitrate (E251 or E252). It may be these additives which upset you rather than the meat itself.

• If you are allergic to chicken, you may find eggs and other poultry affect you. Some people who cannot eat chicken, apparently can tolerate capons (male chickens).

• Chicken and other poultry which have been frozen or water-chilled will most probably contain added water and sodium polyphosphate E450(c) but the added water (if it is below a certain amount) will not be declared. E450(c) acts as water retainer and must appear on label; if you see it, take it for granted that water has also been added. Ham and bacon may also have E450(c) and water added.

• Most animals and poultry bred to be eaten are continuously given antibiotics in their feed not only to ward off infection and disease but also to act as growth promotors. The majority of them (80% of cattle) are also given hormone inplants to encourage growth. Although theoretically the animal should not be slaughtered while the hormones are still in their system, this is not always possible to control and residues may remain. Unfortunately it will be impossible for you to discover whether the meat you buy has residues of antibiotics and hormones unless your butcher buys meat from a farmer who refuses to use these drugs (very few do not use them).

# Nuts

Twelve people out of my survey of 230 said that nuts in some form gave them trouble. Seven blamed peanuts (although they are a vegetable, not a member of the nut family) for causing eczema (twice), asthma (twice), arthritis, indigestion and headache (once).

Anne wrote this lament about peanuts: 'I have little to contribute other than the discovery after many, many years that peanuts poison me. Time was when I ravished and laid waste bowls of nuts during over-long and too frequent cocktail parties. For the past 20 years I have eaten them very infrequently but whenever I have, I suffered acute indigestion; later this became chronic indigestion until about six years ago I became ill within 30 minutes of consuming only six peanuts. My symptoms were heavy sweating, chronic gripey stomach pains and the feeling I would pass out if I did not get air immediately (witnesses say I turn pale grey rather than white). Most times I was not sick but felt perfectly awful for about two hours. This effect can be most embarrassing to one's host not to mention oneself so I now avoid peanuts and peanut oil like the plague.'

Four people said all nuts caused eczema twice and headache and asthma once. One lady from Wembley said walnuts caused an attack of asthma within minutes.

**How to help yourself with nuts.** Think of nuts individually: peanuts, cashew nuts, hazel nuts, brazil nuts and so on.

• If you buy nuts in their shells and open them yourself, you can be sure it is the nut itself which may be causing the trouble; and not any additives.

• Watch out for packed nuts which may contain other ingredients and additives. Roasted peanuts and cashew nuts may contain the flavour enhancer monosodium glutamate (621) for instance.

• If you buy packed nuts from a shop, you can check what the ingredients are from the label. But beware of eating them from a bowl in a pub, restaurant or friend's house with no such identification.

• If you are allergic to peanuts, avoid peanut butter and oil.

• Coconuts and coconut oil may cause trouble to some people. Coconut oil may only be disclosed as vegetable oil.

• Almonds and peanuts contain salicylates (see p.76).

## Vegetables

Beetroot, celery, carrots, onions, potatoes and tomatoes: all these vegetables were quoted as one of the causes of somebody's symptoms. Beetroot was the cause of a 55 year old lady's migraine and one little boy's eczema. Celery caused a lady's face and body to swell and carrots caused migraine in two cases. Onions brought on hayfever type symptoms which lasted 24 hours.

Potatoes made one lady's hands come out in a rash so now she cannot peel them without wearing gloves; and potatoes also brought on asthma in two cases.

Mary wrote this about her son's asthma: 'Even though my son is now 41 years old, I am unable to peel potatoes, cook them or put them on a plate for myself without bringing on an asthmatic attack in him. He is unable to eat crisps, potatoes in any shape or form or even walk past a chip shop without being affected.' Mary discovered the cause of her son's asthma when he was a toddler at kindergarten. 'One day each week he had to take a potato to school and the teacher would cut it up for him to dip into water colour paints to make a pattern on a piece of paper. Each week I received a phone call to take him home as he had collapsed. When he stopped taking that lesson, all was well with him.'

Soya beans were mentioned once by a lady from Worcestershire: 'I discovered the soya bean reaction only after some time. I had been suffering from headaches that varied in the extent of their severity and my doctor referred me to an optician but the headaches continued. I happened to be comparing notes with a close friend who is a life-long sufferer from migraine and she told me that she could not tolerate any of the heavy pulses on account of their fat content. I thereupon cut the soya out of my diet and my headaches ceased. Some months later I ate some soya to test the reaction and sure enough I was again attacked by a fiendish sick headache. I have never touched a soya bean since.'

Tomatoes were reported as one of the causes of two people's migraine and two people's eczema. Hyperactive children are advised to test tomatoes as well as cucumber as both contain salicylates (see p.76).

A study of 88 children suffering from migraine showed that 13 children could not eat tomatoes, seven could not eat soya, four potatoes, three carrots, two peas and two lentils. Leeks, lettuce, cucumber, cauliflower, mushrooms and runner beans each caused migraine once in different children.[2]

**Soya beans** are commonly used as a meat substitute. They contain many of the same proteins (but not all) plus good amounts of iron and vitamins. Processed (textured) soya beans are manufactured to look like meat and this is often mixed with conventional tinned meat products or sold canned without meat to be used to make meatless stews, cutlets and so on. Dried textured soya has to be reconstituted with water. It is either sold plain or mixed with other ingredients in various meat-like recipes like curry and bolognaise sauce. If you buy processed soya products, check on the label to see what else has been added. Soya flour, oil and bran are also available but usually only from health shops, For details of soya milk, see p.154.

**Frozen vegetables** are a good alternative if you cannot buy fresh. They do not usually contain any added ingredients but always check the label before you buy.

**Canned vegetables** vary in what may have been added to them. Some have salt and maybe sugar added. These include sweet corn, mushrooms, asparagus and tomatoes. If you can eat these vegetables and do not mind salt and sugar added, they may be useful to stock your emergency cupboard.

Tinned green-looking vegetables like peas usually have colouring added as well as preservatives. An alternative process may eliminate the use of colour but still includes a preservative, sulphur dioxide (E220) with possibly sodium hydroxide (E524) and monosodium glutamate (621) added. Avoid all these.

Watch out for tins containing mixed vegetables if you feel you may be allergic to any particular one and check the ingredients on the label if the vegetable comes in a sauce, e.g. potato salad. Baked beans made by Heinz contain beans, tomatoes, sugar, salt, modified starch (made from corn), spirit vinegar and spices. Other brands may include these ingredients but some include more. If you are not allergic to any of these ingredients, include a couple of tins as a stand-by in your cupboard. They make a nutritious, tasty snack and most children seem to enjoy them. Heinz states on the label that the product is free from artificial colour and preservative.

**Dried vegetables** contain preservatives and maybe colouring. Avoid them.

**Bottled vegetables** are usually pickled. Some contain preservatives and colouring, others do not. Choose carefully.

**Vegetable oils.** If you use vegetable oil for frying or in salads for instance, use one which consists of one vegetable only. Blended vegetable oils do not say which vegetables or nuts they come from.

**Hydrogenated vegetable oil** is oil which has been treated with hydrogen at a certain temperature and pressure in the presence of nickel. This converts liquid oil into a more solid form and helps prevent rancidity.

**Hydrolysed vegetable (plant) protein** comes from soya or other vegetable protein and is used in many savoury foods, e.g. soups, stock cubes. Hydrolysis breaks down the protein into smaller compounds and results in a coloured mixture with a pronounced flavour. Although no monosodium glutamate (621) is added, in theory by hydrolysis, glutamic acid which is naturally present in vegetables may fix onto free sodium compounds and so form monosodium glutamate. If you have symptoms from monosodium glutamate or other flavour enhancers (620–637) you might check whether these are caused by hydrolysed vegetable protein too. See also p.162.

**How to help yourself with vegetables.** Consider each vegetable separately, e.g. cauliflower, peas, beans, mushrooms.

• If you suspect one, test it by eating it with foods you know do not affect you.

• It may not be the vegetable itself which causes a reaction but a fertilizer, fungicide or pesticide which has been absorbed into it. Over 97 per cent of all vegetables are sprayed with one or more pesticides and several applications may be used for one crop.[3] A survey conducted by the Association of Public Analysts showed that almost a third of vegetables sold in high street shops carried some pesticide contamination.[3] It will probably be impossible for you to discover if a particular pesticide, fungicide or fertiliser is the cause although you may find eating organically grown vegetables a safer bet.[4]

• Wash all vegetables thoroughly.

• Remember crisps are made from potatoes but they also contain other ingredients and additives as well.

• If potatoes in a restaurant affect you but not at home, it may be because they have added whiteners to stop them discolouring.

• Vegetables are full of vitamins and minerals but if you over-cook them, much will be lost. It is better to steam or bake vegetables than to boil them but try eating them raw, except for potatoes which must be cooked and all dried beans including kidney beans which must be boiled first (not just baked in the oven with a casserole for example).

• Some vegetables contain salicylates (see p.76).

• When you buy frozen or canned vegetables, check their labels for additives.

• Use vegetable oils made from one type of vegetable.

## Storage

Plastic containers can give off fumes (you need only open one and smell it to convince yourself). If you feel this might upset you, store food in glass containers. Also do not use plastic wrapping: use grease-proof paper or aluminium foil instead.

Notes
1 *Not All In The Mind,* Dr Richard Mackarness, Pan Books, 1980.
2 *Is Migraine Food Allergy?* J. Egger et al, The Lancet, 15 October 1983.

3  A *Friends of the Earth* report for the Pesticides Action Network (UK) March 1984.

4  Organically grown fruit and vegetables are cultivated without the use of artificial fertilisers or chemical pesticides, herbicides and fungicides. The Safeway chain of food stores stocks a range of organically grown fruit and vegetables throughout the UK. Waitrose has also been selling some organically grown vegetables in selected stores and hopes to get more of these goods into more of its shops in the future. There is no free, comprehensive list of suppliers of organically grown fruit and vegetables but *The Organic Food Guide* edited by Alan Gear, published by Henry Doubleday Research Association, price £2·50 + 50p p&p includes a large list of outlets in England, Scotland and Wales. *Organic Farm Foods* publishes a free list of shops and wholesalers whom it supplies with organic products; and *Action Against Allergy* may also be able to tell you about a shop in your area. If you want to grow your own fruit or vegetables using only natural means, *the Soil Association* has a list of books on how to go about it; the books can be bought from the Association by post. It also publishes a document on organic growing standards together with a permitted list of what should and should not be used for £1. (Addresses in Appendix 1).

5  *Food Additives*, Erik Millstone, Penguin Special, 1986.

# 6

# Milk and other dairy products

## Cows' milk

Out of 230 people who said they were allergic to certain foods, nearly one third said that cows' milk was the cause, or one of the causes, of their allergy (see Appendix 3). If you have read through the first few chapters of this book, especially Chapter 2 where different types of allergy are described, you will have seen many examples of cows' milk causing problems. Here is another one which goes to prove my mis-quotation: the proof of the food allergy is in the eating.

Jean writes: 'My younger son, Paul who is now nine, suffers from asthma, eczema, migraine, hyperactivity and also hair falling out. One day he sat on my lap crying "Please help me Mummy, I don't want to be the way I am." Medicine relieved the problem but did not cure it. Then I heard about goats' milk. Fortunately I live near a farm and started him on the milk with amazing results. His hair grew again, the eczema healed without the cream, his personality changed almost overnight and he slept through the night for the first time in months. At Christmas I was unable to get goats' milk so put him on skimmed milk and for the first week he was covered in a rash. Then it disappeared so I thought all was well. After a while all the old symptoms returned so I took him back to the doctor and asked for a letter to take to the dairy for priority goats' milk and got it. Like magic he returned to normal.'

Having found goats' milk helped her younger son, Jean then thought about how it might help her older son. He had been under hospital supervision for most of his life with ear, nose and throat trouble and had had four ear operations for fluid in the middle ear. 'Eventually they (the hospital) said it was the London air and there was no cure unless we moved. Here we are now in Margate and in the past two months he has had fluid again. The medicine he had again relieved it but did not cure it. Is it food allergy, I wondered, and also put him on goats' milk. Within a week, his ears cleared and he can now hear again.'

Jean found the answer by using goats' milk instead of cows' and many letters said that goats' milk was a satisfactory alternative. However some people may also be allergic to goats' milk so consider this if you change over and test it out. Sheep's milk and soya milk may also be good alternatives. More details of these are given later in this book.

Pat found that rotating different kinds of milk helped her young daughter. After discovering the child was allergic to cows' milk, she was given a soya substitute. Pat continues: 'But after two years of large amounts daily (as recommended by a hospital dietician), it seems that her asthma started with an allergy to the soya. I eventually went to a very good allergy doctor (private) who sorted out her allergies and, having a rest from soya, she tolerates a rotation diet of goats' milk, soya milk (she still can't tolerate the Formula S baby food but can take ordinary soya cartons) and Carnation milk. Apparently 60% of milk allergic people can tolerate butter and Carnation milk although it is wise to keep these in rotation to avoid sensitivity. Since I started this regime of rotation, my daughter has not had any asthma (to speak of) and that was nine months ago. Previously she was ill every two to three weeks.'

**What is in cows' milk.** By law, nothing may be added (except in the case of dried and sweetened condensed milk: see below) but the milk is treated in various ways to keep it fresh. These different treatments are identified by the different coloured aluminium tops on the bottles; or by a full description on the carton.

**Silver top (pasteurized)** is heated to about 72°C for 15 seconds: this kills off any disease-carrying bacteria. Silver top lasts two to three days in a cool place, four to five days in a fridge.

**Gold top** is similar to silver top but comes from cows of the Channel Islands and South Devon breeds. These cows produce a richer milk which is higher in fat content.

**Red top (homogenized)** is pasteurized milk which has had its fat globules broken up mechanically and distributed throughout the milk so they no longer form a creamy surface at the top of the bottle. Red top will last two to three days in a cool place, four to five days in a fridge.

**Green top** is neither pasteurized nor homogenized. Green top with a gold stripe is Channel Island milk which is also untreated. Both must be labelled 'untreated milk' and can only be obtained directly from farmers licensed to sell it. They will last one to two days in a cool place, three to four in a fridge. They are not considered suitable for young children as although the cows are tested regularly for infections, this does not happen evey day so disease could be passed on.

**Longlife (UHT)** is sold in cartons and is usually homogenized milk which is heated to about 130°C for one second and then packed into containers to protect it from light and oxygen. Longlife will keep for several months without refrigeration if unopened; it has an expiry date on the carton. When opened it lasts the same time as fresh milk.

**Sterilized** comes in a plastic bottle with a blue top or a long necked bottle with a metal top. It is prepared from homogenized milk, bottled and then heated to about 120°C for 20 to 60 minutes. As the milk loses up to half of some of its vitamins during this process, use Longlife instead. Sterilized milk will keep two to three months if unopened.

**Skimmed** milk is often sold as instant dried powder and has to be reconstituted with water. Most of its fat has been removed together with Vitamins A and D. Longlife (UHT) cartons of skimmed and semi-skimmed milk are now sold in the shops and you may also be able to buy them bottled (skimmed milk: blue and silver top; semi-skimmed: red and silver top) from your milkman.

**Dried powder milk** may contain other ingredients apart from milk such as soya fat, glucose syrup (made from corn), emulsifiers and other additives. Look at the label before you buy.

**Evaporated and sweetened condensed milk** is concentrated at low temperatures and then sterilized in cans at 115°C for 15 minutes. Vitamin D may be added. It will keep unopened for many years. Sweetened condensed milk has sugar added.

**If you are concerned about antibiotics in milk,** you need not be. It is highly unlikely that your milk is regularly contaminated. Twenty years ago, you might have been right to be concerned as the level was deemed sufficiently high for a Government White Paper to be issued about it. Now milk is tested regularly and farmers are fined heavily if antibiotics are found in their supply. That is not to say that a small amount may not get through the system. Milk samples are taken every day from each supplier but only one sample may be tested during a week and then only after that milk has gone into the main supply. Some samples are tested daily. There is a chance therefore that milk containing antibiotics from one or more cows may go undetected. The Milk Marketing Board says that on average one or two testings out of a thousand show antibiotics in the milk. However risks are further lessened because the milk is usually mixed with other milk in giant vats containing 25,000 to 30,000 gallons so the contaminated milk is very much diluted. It is impossible for you to discover if antibiotics in milk are the cause of occasional symptoms although if you are allergic to antibiotics, you may become suspicious. The Milk Marketing Board says that it has received only two reports of allergy due to antibiotics in milk and these were found during clinical testing where the level of antibiotics was much higher than has ever been found in the testing of milk. Dairy cows are not fed additional hormones.

**How to help yourself with cows' milk**
• While discovering if cows' milk is the cause of your allergy, eliminate all cows' milk products. These include cream, yogurt, cheese, butter, ice cream (both dairy and ice cream containing 'non milk fat') and milk chocolate. Components of milk used in manu-

factured foods are: whey, curd, lactose and casein (caseinate). Food additives which may be based on these components are: E270, E325, E326, E327, E472(b) and 478. Look out for these ingredients on labels: they appear on many. For instance whey is found in many margarines or in powdered form in biscuits.

• Try as an alternative: soya, goats' or sheep's milk. These drinks are described later in this book. If you wish to substitute soya milk in a baby's or young child's diet, you must consult your health visitor or the dietician at your local hospital to ensure your child is getting enough calcium and vitamins. For babies under six months, all milk should be specially modified.

• If you are allergic to cows' milk, the Milk Marketing Board says you may be able to tolerate some milk products like butter or hard cheese. Re-introduce these individually into your diet and test them out. You may also be able to tolerate Carnation evaporated milk.

• Some people who are allergic to cows' milk, cannot eat beef and other beef products.

If you feel you can tolerate cows' milk sometimes, here are a few points to consider:
• Red top (homogenized) milk may be easier to digest than silver, gold or green tops as the fats have been broken down. Similarly skimmed milk, which has almost all its fat removed, may also help.
• Heating milk changes its composition so you may find that Longlife milk which has been heated to a very high temperature suits you better.

## Cream

Cream is made from the butterfat of cows' milk and must have nothing added to it. The exception is whipped cream (cream that has already been whipped as opposed to whipping cream) which may contain sugar and stabilizers E401 and E455.

## Butter

A 250 g pack of butter (equivalent to the old half pound) contains the cream of ten pints of milk. Salt, lactic acid cultures and food colourings: annatto (E160b), carotene (E160a) and turmeric, are allowed to be added to butter by law although most manufacturers do not add colouring. Brands of butter, which do not contain added colouring, are: Anchor, Kerrygold, Lurpak, Countrylife, Longboat, Cottage, and Wheelbarrow. Supermarket own brands include: International, Safeway, Waitrose, English Dales (ASDA), Sainsbury, Presto, Marks & Spencer, Sunshine, Finefare, Mace, Summergold, Wavyline.[1] Colouring should be disclosed on the packet if it is used.

## Butter versus margarine

Margarine is made from a variety of processed oils. Some margarines contain only vegetable oil but others include animal or fish oil. The label on the packet should tell you whether vegetable or animal oil is used. If you are in any doubt, check with the manufacturer, particularly if you suspect you are sensitive to certain oils, e.g. grain oils. Salt, emulsifiers (E322, E471) colouring, usually annatto (E160b) or sometimes carotene (E160a), flavouring and water are added as well as vitamins A and D. Whey (a by-product of milk) is often added and sometimes antioxidants are used. Margarine is meant to look and taste like butter – or even better according to the margarine advertisements.

   Which do you choose? If you can tolerate butter, go for butter; but in moderation. There are fewer substances added to it and therefore less ingredients and additives to suspect. If you cannot take butter, use margarine without whey or any milk in it. You may have to visit a health shop in order to find such a product; or try Tomor margarine which does not contain any milk or whey but does contain added salt, colouring (annatto, code number E160b) and flavouring.

## Yogurt

Most yogurt in the UK is made from cows' milk although in many other countries ewes' (sheep) or goats' milk is used. It is usually made from concentrated skimmed milk which has been pasteurized and homogenized and called low fat on the container but it may be made from any mixture of whole, skimmed, or dried milk.

There must be no antibiotics in the milk which makes yogurt; if there are, the bacteria which create the yogurt will not grow. So each consignment of milk is tested before the starter culture of bacteria is introduced. There are two ways to mature yogurt: in the pots in which it is sold (when it has a 'set' appearance) or in large vats from which, when ready, it is transferred into small containers (this method makes the yogurt have a thinner consistency).

Plain yogurt does not usually contain any additional ingredients although some may have vitamins A and D added; this will be disclosed on the pot. Any other ingredient or additive should be listed on the pot so check before you buy.

Plain yogurt is reported to have healing properties on open wounds such as ulcers and sores. It has also helped eczema suffers. It should be applied directly onto the affected part. I do not know whether it works but it may be worth a try.

Fruit or nut yogurts usually contain other things besides the yogurt and fruit or nuts specified; and in some cases not much fruit or nuts anyway. If you are allergic to any particular fruit or nut, bear this in mind when you eat it in a yogurt.

When research on this book started in 1983, almost all fruit yogurt commercially produced in Britain contained additives. Only a few imported from France contained none. Now, some manufacturers have appreciated the fact that the consumer wants a more natural product and they are bringing out additive-free yogurt. However despite this, colouring, preservatives, stabilizers and emulsifiers are still commonly used but these are disclosed on labels. If gelatin (made from beef bones) or starch (made from corn or wheat) is used, these should also be itemised. Watch out for claims that a particular yogurt contains 'no preservatives' when it may well contain colouring or other additives. Additive-free yogurts often sit on shop shelves next to ones containing ingredients you may wish to avoid and they both may be made by the same manufacturer. Always check the list of ingredients before you buy.

# Cheese

If cows' milk is the cause of your allergy then cheese may affect you similarly but cheese should be considered separately from milk as it contains other ingredients. Cheese, on its own, seems to cause most trouble to people who suffer from migraine or headaches. This may be because cheese contains tyramine which is thought to produce migraine attacks (see p.77).

**What is in cheese.** Cheese is usually made from cows' milk although you can quite easily buy goats' and sheep's cheese. A starter culture of special bacteria and rennet (a liquid extract from a calf's stomach) or other enzymes (see p.169) is added to the milk causing the curd (solid part of milk) to gradually separate from the whey (liquid part). Salt is added during the process and calcium salts may be added at certain times of the year when the calcium content of the milk is lower than normal. The separated curd can be eaten fresh, e.g. cottage cheese, or formed into shapes to ripen and mature.

White hard cheeses contain no colouring but other hard cheese may be coloured with E160a, E160b, E160e and E161g – see Appendix 2 for their full names. The rind may contain virtually any colouring. Blue veined, Provolone and Feta can be coloured with E140 and E141 and Mozzarella with E171. Sage cheese can be coloured with several green colours. The use of colouring should be disclosed on labels.

Preservatives may also be used in cheese. Sorbic acid (E200) is often used in soft cheese (Brie and Lymeswold are examples of soft cheese), rarely in hard cheese. Nitrates and nitrites (E249–E252) are not allowed in Cheddar, Cheshire, Grana-padano or Provolone type cheese or soft cheese but may be found in the following: Danablu, Danbo, Edam, Gouda, Havarti, Samsoe, Tilsiter, Limburger, Saint-Paulin, Svecia, Esrom, Herrgardsost, Hushallsost, Norvegia, Maribo, Fynbo, Amsterdam, Leidse (Leyden) and Friese. Preservatives should be disclosed on labels. Soft cheese may also contain emulsifiers.

Wrapped cheese which contains any colouring, preservative or emulsifier must be labelled with this information. So watch out for it if you think any of these may affect you. If the cheese is sold at the counter, there should be a notice next to it indicating any added ingredients. Except at the major supermarket chains, my experience is that this notice is most unlikely to be displayed. Wrapped cheese may well be a safer bet if you are concerned about its ingredients and according to a recent report may in fact be fresher than its unwrapped counterpart.[2]

Processed cheese and cheese spread are made by melting cheese, usually with emulsifying salts. They may contain the same ingredients as other cheese plus gelatin, additional colourings and preservatives. Look at the labels to see which ones.

**How to help yourself with cheese.** If you are allergic to cows' milk and cheese, try goats' cheese (the French version is called chevre) or sheep's cheese (pecorino or rochefort).

• You can buy cheese with a vegetable rennet. It is often called 'kosher' cheese and can be obtained from delicatessen and health food shops. Some large supermarkets are also beginning to stock it.

• Keep cheese in a cool place, a larder or your fridge. Wrap it in foil or greaseproof paper to prevent drying out. It should be left out in room temperature for about one hour before serving to allow its full flavour to return.

## Goats' milk

Goats' milk is an alternative to cows' milk and many people have found it a successful substitute. Its fat globules are smaller and so may be easier to digest. However some people have found they are allergic to goats' milk as well.

As goats in the UK do not carry the risk of the same diseases TB and brucellosis as cows do (this may not be the case in other countries), goats' milk is often sold untreated (unpasteurised) but pasteurised goats' milk is now appearing in some shops. Some users feed even small children on untreated goats' milk but doctors and dieticians stress that the milk should be boiled to ensure no other harmful bacteria are passed on. Pasteurised goats' milk does not need to be boiled. If you boil the milk, some of the vitamins will be destroyed so it may be necessary to supplement them in young children who are not getting enough from the rest of their diet: ask your health visitor or local hospital dietician to advise you. Do not give goats' milk, whether or not it is pasteurised, to babies under six months old before consulting your doctor or health visitor: it could be dangerous.

Goats' cream, cheese, yogurt and butter can also be purchased. A list of suppliers is available from the British Goat Society (see address in Appendix 1).

## Sheep's milk

Sheep's milk is an alternative to both cows' and goats' milk. It contains twice as much protein and minerals as cows' and goats' milk and 50 per cent more fat. The comments made above about giving goats' milk to babies and children apply equally to sheep's milk.

Sheep's milk, cheese and yogurt can be obtained direct from local farms or from town suppliers. A list of producers is available from the British Sheep Dairying Association (see Appendix 1 for address).

## Eggs

Eggs are a fairly common cause of food allergy. About 15 per cent of my survey of 230 people said eggs were a cause of their symptoms: you will have read examples in the previous chapters. Eczema and skin complaints were the most common although asthma, cold-like symptoms, headaches and one case of depression were amongst those reported (see table in Appendix 3). Allergy to eggs mostly seemed to coincide with allergy to other foods, often other dairy produce.

**Yellow yolks.** You may wonder why the yellow of your eggs varies in colour. This is caused by the sort of feed hens are given. The yolks become more yellow if the hens are fed maize (corn) or grain coloured with certain carotene dyes: E160c,e,f; E161b,c,e,g,h,i (see Appendix 2 for their full names).

Other colourings eg tartrazine (E102) are not allowed to be added to the feed. However, if waste products are fed to the hens for example broken biscuits and these contain tartrazine, then this is permissible.

**How to help yourself with eggs.** You may find you are more sensitive to the white of an egg than to the yolk. This may be because the white contains the protein (albumin) and the protein is often the cause of allergy; or because the white is believed to have a histamine-releasing action (see p.76).

• Eggs more thoroughly cooked like omelette or scrambled egg may affect you less than a soft boiled or fried egg.

• I received two reports of symptoms occurring after eating egg fried in butter or oil: the combination of these two ingredients was thought to be the cause. You might want to bear this in mind.

• Eggs are added to many processed foods, e.g. cakes, pastry and mayonnaise. Watch out for it on labels.

• Albumin (egg protein) is added to many processed foods.

• Lecithin, an emulsifier coded E322, may be made from egg yolk.

• If you are allergic to eggs, you may also react to chicken and possibly other dairy produce but check these out individually.

• There is no difference between brown and white eggs; they just come from different breeds of hen.

**Notes**
1.  List supplied by Butter Information Council.
2 .  *How fresh is fresh,* a Presto Report, Argyll Stores Ltd, April 1984.

# 7

# Wheat, corn and other grains

## Wheat

Skin complaints, wheezing, indigestion, headaches, arthritis, hyperactivity and depression: 41 people (in my survey of 230) said that eating wheat in some form caused one or more of these unwelcome symptoms. Many of these people mentioned that other foods also caused trouble. Seventeen said they were allergic to wheat in general; six said it was the gluten in wheat which caused the problem (see p.75); and 15 people said that only white flour and bread caused their allergy.

You will have read about allergy to wheat elsewhere in this book but here is an example of 'white bread' allergy. Rosemary writes: 'From my early teens (I am now in my middle fifties) I suffered from a very nasty skin complaint which took the form of large raised red rings which were terribly irritating, the more I scratched the bigger they became. I was so ashamed of them: I could not wear a sleeveless dress or bathing suit as they were so unsightly. After approximately three or four weeks they would disappear, only to reappear again within a month or so.

'I did go to my doctor who gave me ointments which did not do any good so I stopped seeing him and just put up with it. About seven years ago I was given the name of a skin specialist. I went to see her and I was told my complaint was caused by additives in food but before I changed my eating habits, she did say that two things that could cause this were tonic water and white bread. I immediately cut out my occasional gin and tonic and started eating only wholemeal bread. From that day I have not had a single occurrence of the complaint and only wish I had known about this before instead of all the trauma I went through.'

# Flour

What is the difference between wholemeal, brown and white flour which makes some people unable to eat all types while others find only white flour and bread affect them badly? All wheat flour, as well as oats, rye and barley, contain gluten. It may be this protein which affects you or another component of the complete wheat.

Over 97 per cent of cereal production in this country is sprayed regularly with one or more pesticides.[1] Residues may remain in the wheat which could be the cause of your symptoms.

**Wholemeal flour** consists of the whole wheat grain including the bran and wheatgerm. Bran is the outer layer of the grain and contains most of the fibre and B vitamins. The wheatgerm is a small part at the base of the grain which contains high levels of protein, fat, vitamins and iron. The bran and wheatgerm often become separated from the rest of the grain during milling and have to be mixed together again afterwards. Wholemeal flour may be coloured with caramel (E150).

**White flour** loses most of the bran, wheatgerm and a lot of vitamins during milling. This turns the flour from brown to white. The milled flour is then usually bleached to further whiten it and flour improvers added[2]. The use of bleaching agents is not declared on labels. The main bleaching agent used is benzoyl peroxide; this is related to the benzoate group of preservatives (see p.166). Flour improvers extend the elastic properties and quicken the development of dough in bread making. Flour improvers have to be disclosed on labels. Two other bleaching agents are chlorine (925) which is only used in cake flour and chlorine dioxide (926). However as these two perfrom another function they are classified as flour improvers and their use must be revealed. Although bleaching agents are not meant to remain in the flour after processing, this may be the reason you cannot eat white flour or its products.

By law white flour has to be fortified with calcium, iron, vitamin $B_1$ and $B_3$ but despite this, there are less of these (except for calcium) and less of other vitamins and minerals in white flour than in wholemeal flour.

**Brown flour** should not be confused with wholemeal flour: it is not the same. It contains less bran and wheatgerm. Theoretically it may even be white bleached flour coloured with caramel (E150) with a certain amount of bran and wheatgerm replaced. However Rank Hovis, a major flour supplier to the bakery trade as well as direct to the consumer, says that it is highly unlikely that brown flour is made from 'bleached' flour and its own flour is not made in this way.

**Self-raising flour** includes raising agents which should be listed on the packet.

**Baking powder** is made from flour and various raising agents. I received a letter from Penny in France saying that the raising agents in flour gave her eight year old son stomach pains and headache. You might suggest it is the flour, not the chemicals, causing these symptoms but Penny says he can eat pancakes and tarts made by herself using plain flour.

# Bread

Most bread sold in Britain is made from wheat flour. White bread, despite the bad press it gets, is still the most popular form of bread in the UK and has been for the last 150 years. Before then, it was considered a delicacy and eaten only by the wealthy. Wholemeal bread, although making a gradual return to the British diet, along with brown bread, still only account for under a quarter of all bread consumption.

White bread is baked with white flour, brown bread with brown flour and wholemeal bread from wholemeal flour. How the flour is processed is described above. Small amounts of rice flour or barley malt flour may be included in all three types of bread.

Wholemeal bread may contain milk, egg, added wheatgerm, oats and extra rice flour but the use of these must be declared in the name of the bread as well as on the list of ingredients of packed bread. Otherwise wholemeal bread can contain most of the ingredients which are allowed in white bread e.g. salt, vinegar, poppy, sesame and caraway seeds, and additives like preservatives and emulsifiers. Bleaching agents and flour improvers e.g. azodicarbonamide (927), potassium bromate (924) and L-cysteine hydrochloride (920) are not allowed in wholemeal bread. The only flour improver allowed in wholemeal bread is ascorbic acid (E300) otherwise known as Vitamin C.

Some breads are known for containing extra ingredients: for instance extra wheatgerm, sodium bicarbonate in soda bread, rye in continental loaves and egg in chollah (plaited loaves).

Granary bread is made from Granary flour which consists of brown flour with added malted wheat flakes. Malted wheat flakes are made from whole wheat grains which have been moistened and allowed to sprout (germinate) for about three or four days when they are heated in a kiln and then flattened into flakes. These give the bread its distinctive taste and texture. Granary flour is a resistered trade mark of Rank Hovis Ltd although other malted wheat flours are produced from either brown or white flour with malted wheat flakes added. Bread made from other brands or malted wheat flour should not be described as Granary though they sometimes are.

Prepacked bread must be labelled with a list of its ingredients and additives but any remaining bleaching agents will not be revealed. Unwrapped bread does not need to be labelled with its ingredients but should have a label, ticket or notice displayed nearby saying which categories of additives have been added eg flour improver, preservative. So if you want to be sure of what you are eating, it may be safer to buy wrapped bread rather than a 'fresh' loaf – unless you get the baker to tell you exactly what ingredients he uses.

## Breadcrumbs

When you buy ready prepared breadcrumbs from a shop check the label carefully. White breadcrumbs will probably not contain any additional additives but 'golden' breadcrumbs may include the yellow food colouring tartrazine (E102) or sunset yellow (E110) or both.

## Pasta and pizza

All pasta is made from wheat. Spaghetti, macaroni and noodles are made from only wheat whilst other pasta like tagliatelle, tortelloni and ravioli include other ingredients. Look at the ingredients on labels carefully if you want to avoid any particular ingredient like egg, tomato or yeast or any colouring, preservative or flavour enhancer which may have been added. Green pasta may be coloured with spinach or artificial colouring may be used. Canned spaghetti, noodles etc., contain many ingredients.

Pizza is now regularly eaten by many British people. It can be bought from many fast food chains specialising in them. Most are made fresh on the premises (see p.175). You can also buy fresh and frozen pizzas in many shops and supermarkets. All their ingredients need to be labelled so check before buying.

### How to help yourself with wheat

• Wholemeal bread may suit you better than white. Remember brown bread is different from wholemeal bread.

• Check out all the ingredients in bread. It may be the milk, eggs, yeast or an additive which is the cause of your symptoms and not the wheat. This may enable you to eat, say, wheat breakfast cereals, but not bread or only certain types of bread.

• Wheat flour goes into the making of rolls, buns, biscuits, pastries and cakes as well as pitta bread, crisp bread, pizzas, pasta like spaghetti and macaroni, pies and matzos (also wafers for Holy Communion).

• Alternatives to wheat flour are corn, potato, millet and rice flour.

• Ryvita and other rye products have been found to be successful

alternatives to bread by many people although rye does contain gluten.
• Many breakfast cereals are made from wheat. Try corn (maize) or rice breakfast cereals instead.
• Starch made from wheat goes into many processed foods. Unfortunately the source of the starch is seldom named so be aware of this fact.
• Semolina is a by-product of wheat.

## Corn (maize)

Five people (out of 230) said that corn was the cause, or one of the causes, of their problems. In one case a young boy became severely ill from migraine of the head and intestine (diagnosed and assessed by doctors); another small boy developed eczema; a lady from Manchester said it was one of the foods which caused her many symptoms; and a fourth said it was one of the causes of her now grown-up daughter's indigestion problems (again this was diagnosed by a doctor). A fifth letter from Surrey said sweet corn gave her son a violent temper and upset co-ordination. This occurred after 20 hours and lasted for 72 hours after eating. 'A dab of juice from a kernel of corn, if he has been eating plenty of it, can produce a welt on the skin within minutes, which is how we discovered it even though it takes so long to come out.'

Corn turns up in your shopping basket in a number of guises. Eaten fresh and called corn on the cob, it is usually boiled. It also comes tinned to be eaten as a vegetable; usually only salt and maybe sugar is added. Frozen corn is available and should contain no additives.

Corn is also used to produce some breakfast cereals. Corn flakes were invented by one of the Kellogg brothers at the end of the last century as a 'health' food. Apparently you were meant to chew it 30 times before swallowing.

Corn flour is used as a thickener for sauces and gravies and you can also buy corn oil. Corn starch can be converted into various forms of syrup which are used in food products as a sweetening agent. These are called glucose syrups in the UK and corn syrups in the USA. Sorbitol (E420) is made from glucose as are the additives 432–436.

If you are allergic to corn (maize), remember that breakfast cereals, flour, vegetable oil, glucose syrup, starch, dextrose and the additives mentioned above may be made from it though not labelled as such. Corn contains salicylate (see p.76).

## Oats

Oats are less commonly eaten in this country but may be found in biscuits and breakfast cereals like muesli and porridge. I received two letters from people who mentioned oats specifically as a cause of their allergy. One included oats with the other gluten products she could not eat (gluten is also found in wheat, barley and rye). The other letter came from a lady in Hastings who singled out oat cakes which she had started to eat in Scotland. 'I ate them without realising my asthma worsened. I took some home for my mother to try, my asthma worsened still further. I continued to eat them as I found a shop locally which sold them. It was not until after I had such severe asthma that I asked my doctor to call (he prescribed Valium which I refused to take) that I considered my diet and stopped taking the oat cakes. Immediately there was an improvement.'

## Barley

Barley contains gluten (see p.75), although this may not be the reason you cannot eat it. If you are allergic to gluten, you may also be allergic to wheat, oats and rye. Malt is made from barley:the seeds are germinated and then roasted.

## Rye

Rye contains gluten. If you are allergic to gluten, you may also be allergic to wheat, oats and barley (see p.75).

## Starch

Starch, food starch, edible starch and modified starch can be derived from maize, wheat, potato, tapioca and sago. Their sources need not be revealed on labels (see also p.168).

## Rice

I received only two reports of rice causing allergy. It caused a small boy to have eczema and provoked a variety of symptoms along with other foods in the second report.

There are basically three types of rice you can buy: brown, white and easy cook rice. Brown rice which has rather a nutty flavour is milled once to remove its outer husk layer. It therefore retains its bran and minerals: phosphorus, sodium, potassium and calcium. White rice is milled to remove the bran: this process turns brown rice into white rice. It is not bleached. Easy cook rice is partially cooked before being milled so some of the goodness from the bran is transferred to the grain before the bran is discarded.

Rice is made into breakfast cereals as well as flour and bran (available from health shops). Many convenience foods, both savoury and sweet, use rice as their main ingredient. Check on the label to see if any of the other ingredients or additives may disagree with you.

## Breakfast cereals

If you are allergic to wheat, corn, rice or oats, check through the list of ingredients on packets of breakfast cereal carefully. People wishing to avoid gluten should choose corn flakes, rice cereals or millet flakes but check there is nothing added which might upset you. Kelloggs says that malt flavouring and extract, which are used in corn flakes and rice cereals, have been shown to be acceptable to coeliac patients (who are sensitive to gluten).

**Notes**
1  A Friends of the Earth Report for the Pesticides Action Network (UK), March 1984
2  Jordans, the flour producers, do not bleach their white flour or add flour improvers.

# 8

# Packaged foods

Do not feel you cannot eat any processed foods. If you find one or several which suit you, continue eating them: you will know that those ingredients and additives (if any) are okay for you. Be careful if you buy what appears to be the same food from a different manufacturer or similar products from the same manufacturer; they may not contain the same ingredients. You will know by reading the label.

For example I have found by experience that my son is not allergic to Bisto gravy. One day he had some gravy away from home and reacted by his typical three to four days of wheezing. What had he eaten that was different to normal? Ah Bisto, I was told. Fortunately I was able to examine the package of gravy. It was not the familiar brown box called 'Bisto Gravy Powder' but a bright red cylinder container called 'Bisto Rich Gravy Granules'. The ingredients were significantly different too, including four more colourings (caramel was in the Powder), two emulsifiers, anti-caking agent, flavour enhancers including monosodium glutamate and two antioxidants. I had discovered the answer as I knew my son is allergic to the flavour enhancer monosodium glutamate (621) and one of the colourings mentioned.

## Ingredients may change

You may find that a product which you have regularly been buying has suddenly been jazzed up in some way. It may just be the packaging which has been redesigned or the ingredients themselves may have changed. Ingredients occasionally change even if the packaging does not. Check regularly: it may seem tedious but you do get used to it. It has become second nature to me now and I find it heartening to see so many shoppers glance at labels and put back anything they do not like the look of.

## Supermarket and other branded products

From July 1986, all processed foods must be labelled with their ingredients and most of their additives. Exactly what has to go on the label is described in Chapter 4.

Because of this and the customers' demand for more additive-free products, some of the large supermarket chains are making serious attempts to reduce the amount of additives used in the food they process. Some of their goods may already be free of additives.

Safeway Food Stores caused a major stir in the middle of 1985 by announcing that it proposed removing 51 additives from its own-label products where possible and practicable. It aimed to start with 26 additives believed to be most frequently implicated in adverse reactions and intended to initially concentrate on those foods eaten in large quantities by children such as soft drinks, ice cream, fish fingers, sausages and jellies.

Waitrose meanwhile has been quietly examining the recipes of all its own label products and by the spring of 1986 intends to sell more than 200 of its products with no additives or only natural ingredients in them.

Marks & Spencer has been selling many additive-free products for several years and says its policy has and always will be to develop additive-free products where possible.

Tesco says it is reducing the amount of additives in its food and is specifically concentrating on the removal of tartrazine (E102) from products such as yogurts and squashes. It has drawn up a list of additives most implicated in terms of allergic responses (colourings, benzoates E210–E218, BHA E230 and BHT E321) with a view to identifying a priority list of products from which to start removing those additives. Tesco claims to stock 400 own label products which are additive free, but many of these are foods which would not contain additives anyway.

Sainsbury's states it is continuing to increase its additive-free range which already includes foods like yogurts, jams and some canned vegetables. It has removed tartrazine (E102) from several products such as ice-cream and fish fingers plus brown FK (154) from its smoked mackerel fillets. It is further looking into whether these and other additives can be eliminated from more products.

The Co-op is also seeking to develop additive-free products. Other supermarket chains are lagging behind but hopefully when they appreciate the success of their competitors in this field, they too will change course.

Heinz has always produced more colour and preservative-free products than other branded goods producers with the exception of specialised manufacturers which tend to produce more expensive items. However many manufacturers may start to change their lines as the demand for additive-free food increases from the public and the supermarkets where they are sold. For example Blue Crest (see p.95) are planning to replace tartrazine (E102) and sunset yellow (E110) with turmeric and annatto (E160b).

Most of the large supermarket chains produce lists of their own label products which do or don't contain certain additives. These can be obtained by writing to the customer services department of the supermarket at the address given on the label of one of its own-brand products. However these lists can possibly be misleading as some will detail colour-free products for example but not necessarily state any other additives used. Your best guide is to read the label on the product you buy.

In this chapter I have given some examples of food you may be buying and what to look out for. While you are trying to find out the cause of your own, or your child's, allergy, go carefully with products which contain many ingredients. It will be very difficult to discover if a particular ingredient amongst many is causing the trouble. If your diary shows you can eat a brand of mayonnaise or ketchup without side effects, however, you can be pretty sure that these ingredients will cause you no harm. For more details of those additives mentioned in this chapter, refer to Appendix 2.

## Baked flour products

**Rolls, muffins, crumpets, scones, waffles, croissants and scotch pancakes** are made with wheat flour and some sort of fat (usually vegetable). Shortening is made from vegetable oil or animal fat. Salt, sugar and sometimes milk may be used and additives such as emulsifiers, preservatives and maybe colouring. Egg and yeast may also be included. Check the ingredients on the label and do not eat anything which includes something to which you think you are allergic.

**Biscuits** come in all shapes and sizes and with many different ingredients. Wheat flour, milk or whey, sugar and eggs may be used. All biscuit packets are labelled. Many biscuits like shortbread and rich tea biscuits do not contain additives but orange and other coloured cream biscuits may use the colours tartrazine (E102), sunset yellow (E110), amaranth (E123) plus more and some biscuits may contain antioxidant.

**Chocolate biscuits** should be considered separately from other biscuits as it may be the chocolate and not the rest of the ingredients which is causing the trouble (see p.134).

**Cakes** bought unwrapped need not declare their ingredients so be on your guard as to what they contain. They may appear to be the same as those you make at home but this may not be the case. Wrapped cakes must list their ingredients.

Why not make your own? Use any sponge recipe and adapt the ingredients to suit yourself. For instance use butter instead of margarine or the other way around if you cannot tolerate milk. Remember that some margarines contain milk and other additives. Alternatively use vegetable oil. Exchange carob powder for cocoa powder if you cannot eat chocolate or squeeze fresh orange or lemon juice into the sponge mixture to make your own flavours. With a little effort you can provide a delicious cake for yourself and your family and have the satisfaction that it contains exactly what you want it to. Food Watch (address in Appendix 1) sells many substitute ingredients with hints on how to use them.

Compare the ingredients you use to make your own with those of a shop bought cake. Cupcakes bought at a supermarket contain: sugar, flour, water, skimmed milk powder, glucose syrup, animal and vegetable fat, egg white, fat-reduced cocoa, egg, dextrose, flavouring, salt, emulsifier E471, glycerine, colours E102, E110, E122, E124, E142, E155: no less than six colourings.

Cheesecake, bought at a well known chain, which prides itself on avoiding as many additives as possible, had listed as its ingredients: Medium fat soft cheese, sugar, egg, margarine, sultanas, wheatflour, dried skimmed milk, flavouring, emulsifiers E475, E471, lemon oil, salt, colours E102, E110.

In both these examples, colouring, unknown flavouring and emulsifiers were used which would not have been if you had baked them at home.

**Cake ingredients** like cherries, marzipan and flavourings can contain colouring and other additives which may disagree with you. A brandy flavouring spotted on a supermarket shelf contained no less than four food colourings. Make your cake with fresh ingredients and flavours taken from natural foods.

**Cake mixes.** What I have said about shop bought cakes applies equally to cake mixes. Read the labels on cake mixes and if they do not contain colour, they may include preservative and almost certainly some sort of emulsifier. I unashamedly repeat what I have said in the previous paragraphs: make your own. It is not much more trouble to use your own recipe of flour, sugar and fat instead of the mixtures obtained from packets.

# Chocolate

Twenty-nine people said that chocolate was the cause, or one of the causes, of their allergy. Thirteen suffered from migraine, five from asthma, four from eczema or skin rashes and one from arthritis, stomach complaint and depression. Chocolate made four children hyperactive.

Here is one such case reported by the Colchester & District Allergy Group: 'Nicky, a little boy of seven years, had behaviour problems. Out of character, he would become increasingly naughty, even cruel to his baby sister. This would get worse and worse until he would have a shaking attack and collapse. His mother was frantic and thought she was going to have a juvenile delinquent on her hands.'

It was suggested to this mother that she eliminate all artificial colouring, flavouring and preservatives from his food and also the chocolate bar which he took every day to school. 'The child started to get better. He maintained this improvement up until New Year's Day when his mother, feeling she had deprived him over Christmas, gave him a chocolate bar as a treat. The next day was dreadful. She was no longer in doubt. Since then, there have been two mishaps: once he won and ate a chocolate bar at a party and a dreadful day followed but the reason was discovered. Another time he was given one chocolate mint and even this caused trouble.'

Chocolate is a well known cause of migraine and headaches. Recently a mother told me her daughter had started taking chocolate to school again and her headaches had reappeared. Needless to say, her daughter will not be eating chocolate anymore. Her teenage son cannot eat chocolate either as it brings him out in spots.

Rosemary told me she felt low for a couple of hours after eating chocolate; and you will have read about other people in this book who have discovered that chocolate is the cause of their symptoms.

**What is chocolate.** Chocolate is made from cocoa which contains caffeine (see p.75). Chocolate is also believed to have a histamine-releasing action (see p.76). Whether symptoms are caused by these or other reasons has yet to be proved. Plain and milk chocolate bars do not have to disclose their ingredients in full nor do any other chocolate products.

If you are allergic to chocolate, you will not be able to eat any food with cocoa or chocolate in it. Try carob instead. You can buy it as a bar or in powder form from most health shops. It tastes very similar to chocolate although carob bar is sweeter unless you buy the 'no added sugar' variety. Used as an ingredient in home-made cakes and puddings, I doubt if you can tell the difference.

## Crisps and other savoury snacks

Crisps are made from potatoes which are fried in vegetable oil, sometimes hydrogenated vegetable oil (see p.108). Plain salted crisps use a lot of salt and most contain an antioxidant, either BHA (E320) or BHT (E321) (see p.168). Flavoured crisps like cheese and onion, salt and vinegar, and prawn often contain flavourings which are not individually disclosed and flavour enhancers usually monosodium glutamate (621) or sodium inosinate (631). Savoury snacks made from wheat or corn (maize) may contain other ingredients plus all these additives and colouring too. A few do not; search them out.

## Honey

Two people told me they were allergic to honey. A lady from Hastings said it caused her to develop 'giant urticaria' (red lumps on the skin). She reports: 'I went on a diet, stopped eating honey and as a result the urticaria has miraculously disappeared.' A second lady reported that honey, along with cola and the yellow colouring tartrazine (E102) made her son have diarrhoea.

Honey is a form of sugar and contains very small amounts of vitamins and minerals. It is sold with nothing added to it; if something is added it cannot be called honey, but could be called, for instance, honey spread (and any extra ingredient or additive must be disclosed). Honey is often heat treated to create a thinner consistency so that it becomes easier to spread.

It may be a suitable substitute for sugar but is just as fattening and bad for your teeth. Some people claim it has healing properties if applied directly to wounds and grazes. I do not know whether this is true: it seems a sticky way to deal with things.

# Jam

Many manufacturers and supermarkets now produce jams which do not contain preservatives or colouring. Pectin (E440a) and citric acid (E330) are sometimes added. Select jams carefully when you buy as those with artificial additives often sit side by side with their natural sisters. Jam contains a lot of sugar so if you are trying to lose weight, reduce the amount you eat. Spreading jam more thinly is a good way to start.

# Ice cream

The majority of commercial ice creams sold in the UK are made with milk, sugar, vegetable fat, emulsifiers, stabilisers and contain colouring. This applies to most brands of fruit flavoured and chocolate ice cream. Vanilla ice cream may, or may not, be coloured: check on the label. More additive-free ice creams are appearing in shops so watch out for them. If you cannot tolerate milk, choose water ices (called sherbet in the USA, sorbet in France) if you can find a brand which contains no additives. A few do exist but they are liable to be expensive. Try making your own ice creams and water ices.

# Jellies

Jellies are made of sugar, gelatin and lots of colouring. Gelatin comes from cows' bones. The colouring used depends on the type of jelly – orange, strawberry, lemon and so on but all use them. If the jelly is yellow, orange or green, it is almost certain to include tartrazine (E102) or sunset yellow (E110), and if it is red amaranth (E123). Some brands include the juice from the fruit described, others do not. There is no goodness in jelly – I advise you and your children to avoid it.

# Puddings

Look carefully at the label when buying shop prepared puddings, desserts, custards and mousses; whether they are ready to eat, frozen or those which have to be mixed with milk or other liquid. They may contain milk (or whey), eggs, starch (made from wheat) and sugar, as well as colourings, preservatives and emulsifiers.

Try making your own desserts. Whip up some cream (if you can take milk) and mix your own fresh fruit into it. Yogurt (goats' or sheep's if you cannot eat cows') mixed with nuts or fruit is very tasty. You may need a little brown sugar or honey to sweeten it. Sprinkle a little grated chocolate or carob on top to entice the children.

Of course fresh fruit on its own makes an excellent 'after' and if you cut it up into small slices or pieces will often be more appealing to children than if the fruit is served whole. If you are going through a testing phase, serve only one fruit at a time (see Chapter 5 on fruit).

## Salt

Household salt is sodium chloride. Your body needs sodium to regulate the amount of fluid (water) it retains and to help in muscular and nerve functions. However many medical experts believe too much sodium can damage your health due to a link between salt and high blood pressure. Government and professional bodies in many countries have recommended a reduction in salt intake. Most people, both adults and children, eat at least twice as much salt as they need so you are unlikely to have a deficiency even if you reduce your consumption. Cramps in your muscles may be a result of having too little salt in your diet but this is not necessarily the cause.

Salt is a preservative as well as a flavouring and has been used to preserve meat and fish for thousands of years. Anti-caking agents are added to table salt to make it flow more easily: they are named on labels.

If you want to cut down on your salt consumption: do not sprinkle it onto your food at the table; reduce the amount you use in cooking; and stop eating salty foods like bacon, ham, sausages, kippers, smoked fish, salted butter, pickles and crisps.

# Sauces and relishes

When you visit your supermarket or grocery, a whole range of sauces, relishes and ketchups line the shelves to entice you. All look appetising and are brightly coloured; usually artificially. They may also contain preservatives, emulsifiers and stabilizers; some contain modified starch to bulk out the product. Here are some examples of what to look for. I have not covered everything. Always check the labels: if you feel you can eat the ingredients, do not feel ashamed to buy the product. This book is intended to help you, not give you more work than is necessary.

**Tomato ketchup** may contain preservatives and occasionally colouring. Heinz tomato ketchup contains tomatoes, sugar, spirit vinegar, salt and spices and is guaranteed free from artificial colour and preservatives. Other brands may also not contain preservatives or colouring but may add flavouring which is not fully described.

**Salad dressing** can easily be made at home with ingredients with which you are already familiar. Oil, vinegar and a little salt and pepper is all you need. I make enough to last for several weeks. The oil will separate from the vinegar but all you need to do is give the container a good shake and they will mix again.

**Salad cream** is made of vinegar, oil, sugar, water, mustard, egg yolk, salt, modified starch, stabilizers and colouring. If you want to avoid the additives, choose mayonnaise instead.

**Mayonnaise** may contain additives; some do not. Shop around for those you feel you can eat. You could make your own but mine always ends up in disaster. So personally I prefer to pay more and make life easier for myself. Remember most contain egg but non-egg mayonnaise is available at health food shops.

**Mint sauce** is always coloured. I have yet to find one that is not. Make your own. Grow some mint in your garden or window box, cut it up finely, mix with vinegar and a little sugar. Leave for at least an hour before use. It might not look as green but it will taste as good.

**Mustard** may contain additives but many brands do not. Watch out for those containing tartrazine (E102) or antioxidants and avoid them.

**Piccalilli** can contain vegetables or additives, especially colourings, which may disagree with you.

**Prawn cocktail sauce** should be treated with caution as it will contain colouring and preservatives. Make your own with tomato ketchup and mayonnaise which are free of colouring and preservatives. Just mix the two together. Fresh lemon juice squeezed on top will give a more tangy flavour. The sauce also makes a good dip for eating with chopped up vegetables like carrot, cucumber, mushrooms, peppers and tomatoes.

## Soup

If you can find the time to make your own soup, do so. Home-made soup is usually tastier and better for you than tinned or packet soups. If you have a blender, soup is made even more appealing especially to children. Cook any vegetable you have and know you can eat in some stock (see below), add some of your own flavouring, for example some herbs, paprika or curry powder and when slightly cool, blend. If you can drink milk and want to, add some to make the soup creamier.

**Stock cubes** should be treated with caution. Most contain the flavour enhancer monosodium glutamate (621). Those, which do not, contain hydrolysed vegetable protein (see p.108). Marmite, a useful flavouring, contains neither but is a yeast extract (see p.143). You can always make your own stock from bones which your local butcher will probably give you at little or no cost; or use the juices from meat you have grilled or roasted which are left in the pan. If you boil vegetables, use the water as stock: it contains many vitamins and minerals drawn from the vegetables.

**Tinned soups** are a handy stand-by. Some varieties do not contain artificial additives although most use a form of starch to thicken them: this may be made from wheat or corn. Some contain milk or whey. Vegetable soups like tomato, mushroom and asparagus tend to contain the least additives but check labels carefully before you buy. Different manufacturers use different ingredients and even similar soups made by the same manufacturer may differ quite considerably in their contents.

I experienced how careful you need to be when I bought a tin of Campbell's tomato soup. The ingredients were tomatoes, wheat flour, sugar, salt, vegetable oil and spices. All things my child could eat. The following week I bought what at first glance seemed the same product. The picture and the printing on the label looked identical. They were not. The first I had bought was ordinary tomato soup; the second was cream of tomato soup. The difference lay not only in the cream and whey powder which had been added but citric acid (E330) and the flavour enhancers monosodium glutamate (621) and sodium inosinate (631) had also been included in the recipe. Heinz Cream of Tomato soup does not contain E330, 621 or 631.

**Dried packet soups** contain more additives than tinned soups so stock your cupboard with tinned soups without additives.


## Sugar

Fifteen people said that omitting sugar from their diet helped reduce their allergy symptoms. One Cleveland grandmother wrote that her worst enemy was sugar: 'It gives me dreadful catarrh and that causes asthma.' Seven people said they suffered from asthma and symptoms relating to their nose and chest whilst two suffered from eczema and two more from stomach complaints. Sugar caused two children to become hyperactive and one person to suffer migraine. One mother thought that sugar had been the cause of her son's bedwetting.

**White sugar,** both granulated and castor, is made from raw sugar beet or cane which is washed and spun to remove its molasses, treated with lime and carbon dioxide and finally with charcoal or resin to remove its colour.

**Icing sugar** is powdered granulated sugar. Calcium phosphate is usually added to prevent it going lumpy.

**Demerara sugar** is either raw cane sugar or white sugar mixed with natural cane molasses. If there are no ingredients on the label, you can assume it is just raw cane sugar.

**Soft brown sugar** is made from white sugar mixed with natural cane molasses.

**Crystal sugar** comes white, brown or coloured. The brown is coloured with caramel (E150), the multi-coloured variety with tartrazine (E102) and other colourings. Avoid these.

**Molasses, black treacle and raw cane sugar** are untreated after being extracted from the plant.

**Glucose (dextrose), fructose and sucrose** are all sugars found naturally in fruits and vegetables.

**Lactose** is a sugar found only in milk (including human milk).

Sugar, in any of the forms mentioned above, is added to many foods such as biscuits, cakes, jams, tinned fruit, ice cream, soft drinks and sweets; and many breakfast cereals are sugar coated. Sugar also goes into many 'savoury' tinned and frozen foods.

Sugar contains no goodness other than it will give you energy but that can be provided by many other more nutritious foods. Molasses and black treacle contain some iron and calcium and traces of other minerals. During the first three months of 1984, on average every person in Great Britain ate over $\frac{1}{2}$ lb. of sugar each week. This amount does not include sugar added to processed foods.[2]

## Sweets

You should try to do without sweets and toffees. They are bad for your teeth and contain no goodness. They contain a lot of sugar which may give you energy but you can get that equally well from a whole lot of other foods. If you must eat sweets, buy non-coloured ones but remember they may contain other additives like anti-oxidants and of course flavourings. Medicated sweets, perhaps containing menthol, may also be coloured and include other ingredients which do not agree with you. Many sweets, which are unwrapped, individually wrapped or sold in transparent packets, will not be labelled indicating what they are made of.

## Yeast and yeast extract

Two asthma sufferers mentioned Marmite (which is a yeast extract product) as causing their symptoms and Liz said it gave her a headache if taken with tea. Gill wrote about her daughter's asthma: 'She became an asthma sufferer at about eight years. We found that Marmite brought on these attacks and anything with yeast extract in it. She is now 29 and has avoided these for a number of years. However she tried Marmite again two years ago and had another severe attack.'

Two asthma sufferers said that yeast was the problem and so did another person who got headaches. Two of the asthma sufferers have had their allergy to yeast confirmed by doctors. Clinical studies have shown that yeast can cause skin disorders.[1]

**Yeast** is an organism, a mould, grown on things like molasses or malt. It goes into many foods. Bread would not rise without it.

**Yeast extract** is an ingredient which goes into breakfast cereals and stock cubes as well as being one of the main ingredients of products like Bovril and Marmite. Some yeast extract products, e.g. Marmite, do not contain any yeast cells as all of them are removed during processing; whereas others, such as Vegemite, do contain yeast cells. Bovril also contains beef extract whilst Marmite contains no meat but is based on vegetable extract. Many supermarkets produce their own brands of both types. Yeast extract products do contain other ingredients so it could be these and not the yeast extract itself which are the cause of the problem.

However yeast extract products are known to contain tyramine and salicylate (see p.76).

**Notes**
1  *Reactions to Food in Adults,* M.H. Lessof in *Clinical Reactions to Food,* John Wiley & Sons 1983.
2  Figure published by the Ministry of Agriculture, Fisheries and Food.

# 9

# Drinks and water

## Water

Four people out of 230 said tap water caused symptoms. Two said
it caused eczema and two complained it caused stomach troubles.
All four also accused other foods of creating symptoms.

Jill from Witney told me about her 19 month old son who had
developed eczema: 'I kept him fully breast-fed until seven months
and gradually introduced him to a wholefood vegetarian diet. He
had bottled spring water to drink as I considered this better than
boiling water. At around his first birthday, he began eating more
solid food and having tap water and his skin worsened. He has not
been clear for the last six months and we discovered he also reacts
to eggs, all bovine products and goats' milk as well as cows' milk.
About six weeks ago, I decided to dispense with tap water and try
bottled water again and the effect was dramatic. His eczema was
reduced by some 75 per cent and he is sleeping better.'

The elements in water vary throughout the country and even
within the area covered by an individual water authority. This is
because it comes from different sources: deep water wells or rivers.
The job of a water authority is to ensure that water is safe to drink
but various trace elements do remain as do some natural minerals.
You need only drink water in different parts of the UK to establish
the fact that it can taste quite different in different places.

**Chlorine** is used extensively to disinfect water against bacteria.
Some people find they cannot tolerate it.

**Fluoride** is artificially added to about 10% of the water supply in Great Britain mainly in the Midlands. That means it is drunk by about six and a half million people. Many medical authorities believe that fluoride is a safe way to protect teeth against decay but one dental surgeon points out that as it strengthens the enamel of children's teeth only when between one to 11 years when all enamel is formed, perhaps other age groups should not be subjected to regular doses. In excess, fluoride can cause mottling of the teeth.

**Nitrates** flow into rivers and underground water from the drainage of agricultural land and from sewage works. East Anglia's water supply contains the highest amounts but there is concern that the level throughout the country is rising.[1] Nitrates can cause problems to some people (see p. 167).

**Lead** from old lead pipes may contaminate your water supply but lead pipes have been banned from use in the plumbing of modern houses. In some areas, water treatment has been adapted to limit the take-up of lead. Run off a bowlful of cold water before you use any for drinking or cooking to help get rid of any lead or sediment.

Water is a necessity of life. You could not survive for more than a day or so without it whilst you can go for weeks and even months without food. Drink plenty of water as it helps all your body functions. In temperate climates such as in Britain, at least two pints a day should be drunk; more if it is hot or you are involved in heavy work.

If you have a headache or feel 'achy', before reaching for a bottle of pills, just drink a pint of water and see if it relieves the symptoms. A cold, damp flannel on the forehead is also an old, and well tried, remedy for headaches. In Europe, drinking and taking the waters at spas has been a popular remedy for many ailments including asthma, stomach disorders and rheumatism, for many centuries.

If you are worried about your water supply and what is in it, ask your local water authority. Get their telephone number from your water bill or from the local directory. Try bottled water instead. It is expensive but may be worthwhile; it will certainly taste different.

Different brands contain different minerals. Water filters which remove chemicals from tap water are obtainable from health food stores and hardware shops.

## Coffee

Eight people said coffee gave them headaches. Janet said coffee was responsible for her bad complexion as well as her headaches: 'I discovered two years ago that I was to a certain degree allergic to coffee and to some extent red wine. Since cutting out coffee almost entirely from my diet, my complexion has more or less cleared of spots and my headaches are much less frequent or severe – what a relief. I have replaced it with weak china tea. Also I am relieved of a strange nauseous feeling after drinking coffee which was how I first hit upon the idea. I can drink the occasional cup of decaffeinated coffee without side effects.'

One other person complained that coffee caused a skin condition and Claudia mentioned that coffee and cheese consumed on the same day 'guaranteed to bring on a severe attack of migraine'. One case of indigestion and one of hyperactivity were reported, and two people suffering from arthritis said coffee was a contributing cause. Mandy started to get arthritis in her hands. As she is a professional knitter, she became very worried about her condition. She cut out coffee along with a number of other foods. Her hands improved. After a couple of months she drank a cup of coffee 'to keep a friend company'. Within 15 minutes she felt weak and washed out. On glancing at herself in a mirror, she found she looked very pale.

**Coffee beans,** which you grind yourself or which are already ground, and all granular and powdered instant coffee have nothing added although they contain caffeine (see p.75) and many other natural substances. Decaffeinated coffee has the caffeine removed. Some coffee mixtures include chicory and maybe malt and barley: these will be disclosed on the label.

**Instant coffee** is made by roasting the beans, grinding them and then percolating them with water to produce a highly concentrated liquid coffee. Granular instant coffee is made either by freeze-drying the liquid (e.g. Gold Blend) or by spray-drying it (e.g. Nescafé, Maxwell House). Powdered coffee is always spray-dried.

**Spray-drying** is a process in which the liquid coffee is blasted by a current of hot air at the top of a metal tower. The water evaporates immediately from the coffee and the humid air is drawn out by ventilators. The coffee particles cool upon falling and are gathered in the lower part of the tower.

**Freeze-drying** is a process in which the liquid coffee is frozen and then ground into tiny fragments. These are placed in a freeze-drying chamber where under vacuum and low heat, the ice crystals evaporate leaving the coffee granules.

**Decaffeinated coffee** is made by extracting the caffeine before the beans are roasted. This may be done by means of a solvent but I am told by Nestlé that their brands, Gold Blend Decaffeinated and Decaf, have the caffeine removed by a water process.

If you stop drinking coffee, you may get withdrawal symptoms of a bad headache and even depression. This should wear off after a couple of days but you might find it preferable to cut down gradually. If you think you are allergic to coffee, try drinking weak tea or maybe herbal tea instead. If you feel caffeine is the reason for your symptoms, try decaffeinated coffee or dandelion coffee and avoid tea, cocoa (chocolate), cola, and fizzy drinks and drugs which contain it. Coffee and tea also contain salicylate (see p.76).

## Cocoa and drinking chocolate

The difference between cocoa and drinking chocolate is that drinking chocolate is sweetened with sugar. Otherwise they both tend to have salt and flavouring added. The flavouring is never described. If you find you are allergic to these drinks, you are probably allergic to chocolate (see p.134).

## Tea

I received two letters mentioning tea. It caused hyperactivity in a small boy and gave Christine symptoms similar to sea-sickness – coffee also produced the same effect in her. Liz told me she cannot drink tea and eat Marmite at the same meal without getting a headache. In a study of 88 children suffering from migraine, seven were found to react to tea.[2] Tea contains caffeine (see p.75) and salicylate (see p.76). On average four cups of tea a day are drunk by every person (including children) in Britain. If you suspect you are allergic to Indian or China tea, try herbal teas instead.

## Cola drinks

Three people said cola drinks gave them symptoms: a rash, diarrhoea and hyperactivity. A friend recently told me her son became very 'jumpy' when he drank cola. My son stopped drinking it five years ago as he wheezed for four days afterwards. Cola drinks are made of carbonated water, sugar, the food colour caramel (E150), phosphoric acid (E338) and flavouring. Some contain preservatives. Only Pepsi Cola discloses it contains extract of cola nut; other cola drinks may contain it but describe it only as a flavouring. Most cola drinks contain caffeine (which is a natural component of the nut). It is the caffeine which gives the drink its 'lift' (see p.75). Diet or slimmers' cola drinks are made in much the same way but the sugar is substituted by artificial sweetener.

If you are a regular cola drinker and you suddenly stop it, you could get caffeine withdrawal symptoms like with coffee, tea or chocolate.

## Fruit juice

See p.100.

## Fruit squash, crush and other fruit drinks

Fifteen people wrote complaining about orange and other fruit drinks and squashes; and another four mentioned blackcurrant drinks. Do not confuse these drinks with fruit juices: they are not the same.

## Orange squash

Here are quotes from some of the letters I received which should
make you think very carefully when choosing drinks for you and
your family. Rose wrote about her husband, now aged 59, who has
suffered from asthma and hayfever for many years: 'He was
advised by hospital doctors that he was allergic to yeast products
and orange and lemon drinks (except pure fruit juices). Even before
the war he was aware that fruit drinks made him wheeze.'

Lynne, like Rose's husband, has suffered from asthma and also
eczema since childhood: 'I have found that I cannot drink orange
squash because of its additives. I soon become breathless.'

Medical research carried out in 1977 revealed that ten out of 14
patients who said they became asthmatic after drinking orange
drinks, did in fact become so.[3]

Jennifer found that cutting out squash has helped her daughter's
eczema but not her asthma. She says: 'I took action five years ago
when I read that eliminating additives might help children who
have eczema. I cut out absolutely everything because at this stage I
had no idea which particular ones were the trouble-makers. My
daughter was always thirsty but within 24 hours of pure food this
problem had gone and after a month her eczema had gone. I kept
her strictly on this diet for two years or so and then gradually
introduced various foods with additives with no recurrence of
trouble. She now eats almost anything and her eczema is hardly
there at all. The only thing still prohibited is orange squash or
anything with orange colouring as these seem to be the worst
trouble-makers. Her asthma did not seem to improve by the diet as
the triggers were probably in the air rather than food. However she
is now 12 and seems to be growing out of that too.'

Vivienne found that squash caused her daughter, now aged five,
other problems: 'From a very early age she had difficulty in
concentrating on the smallest things and was very highly strung.
She then started to have bad sleeping periods when she woke up
screaming and shouting and generally having hysterics. I took her
to see my health visitor who hit on the idea of not giving her any
more orange squash but instead to buy the pure fruit juices

available. By not giving her squash to drink, she has become much more calm and has had no more bad sleep periods. I found that blackcurrant drinks had the same effect as squash so now she drinks nothing but pure fruit juice.'

One of the most interesting revelations which came out of my appeal for people's experience of food causing problems was that drinking squash may be a cause of bed wetting. You will have read about one little girl having this problem in Chapter 2. Another girl who also suffered from this distressing problem was fortunate that her mother realised there might be a connection and eliminated orange squash. She no longer wets the bed and sleeps much more soundly.

## Blackcurrant drinks

One case of eczema, one of eczema with diarrhoea and two of wakefulness at night: these four were attributed to blackcurrant drink. Often called a health drink, it mav not be for you.

Claire wrote: 'I have a little girl who is 22 months. A couple of months ago, she was sleeping very badly. She has never been a good sleeper and goes to bed quite late, about ten, but at that particular time she was waking up two or three times during the night. This was quite usual but she would then take anything up to an hour to go back to sleep again (not usual). Normally I could give her a bottle of juice and she would go straight to sleep again.

'I came to the end of my tether one Monday night. She woke at 2.30 am and was still awake at 4.30 am. I went into my husband crying and she ended up in the middle of us. I visited the health visitor that day. She asked if she drank a lot of juice. I pointed out she drank a lot of blackcurrant drink which had worried me although I was not aware what harm it was doing. She recommended I stop giving it to her immediately.

My daughter had her last drop of blackcurrant drink that Tuesday afternoon. She cried for it that evening and during the night. Wednesday night she had what appeared to be withdrawal symptoms. As she was going off to sleep in my arms, she was twitching and jumping. After three nights, there was a definite improvement. She now wakes only once, sometimes not at all, but she goes straight back to sleep. She actually gets into a much deeper sleep than previously. She now drinks only milk and natural juices and I try to avoid foods with added flavouring and colouring.'

In 1983 a mother mentioned that her child could drink Baby Ribena blackcurrant drink without side effects but not the usual Ribena blackcurrant drink. What was the difference? Baby Ribena does not contain any preservatives, colouring or artificial sweetener wheras Ribena at that time contained the preservative sodium metabisulphite (E223) and the colour amaranth (E123). I asked Beechams, the manufacturer, why there was a difference. I was told Baby Ribena has a shorter shelf life before opening – it may turn brown; and once opened it may not keep as long which is why it is only sold in small bottles. (There is a recommendation by the World Health Organisation not to include unnecessary additives in products designed specially for babies). Preservatives and colouring were added to Ribena (and other brands of blackcurrant drinks) to make them last longer. In 1985 the ingredients of Ribena blackcurrant drink were changed. Natural colouring anthocyanin (E163) is now used and the preservative sodium benzoate (E211) has been added to the existing one sodium metabisulphite (E223) which has been reduced to a quarter of its original level. Ribena 'ready to drink' drinks in cartons do not contain preservatives except for the sparkling variety in cans which uses sodium benzoate (E211). See p.166 for more information on these preservatives.

## What is in fruit squashes and other drinks

Besides the fruit, e.g. orange, lemon, blackcurrant, there is sugar (usually more sugar than fruit) often in the form of sucrose or glucose syrup, artificial sweetener (probably saccharin), fruit acid (maybe citric acid), flavouring, preservatives, stabilizers and colouring. The colours used differ according to the type of fruit drink but most contain one or more of these azo dyes: E102, E110, E123, and E124; other colours may also be used. The preservative is usually sodium benzoate (E211) but again others may be used.

Orange and other citrus squashes need only contain 25 per cent fruit juice (other fruit squashes only 10 per cent) and should be diluted with water. Crush is sold ready to drink and need only

contain 5 per cent fruit juice. Fruit 'drinks' come either concentrated and have to be diluted with water, or are sold already
diluted. They need only contain 10 per cent fruit pulp or fruit juice
(if undiluted), 2 per cent fruit pulp or 5 per cent fruit juice (if ready
to drink).

If you are allergic to fruit squashes and other 'drinks', it could be
the fruit itself causing the trouble or it may be one of the additives
which is the culprit.

## Fizzy drinks

Almost all contain preservatives and most will be coloured. Some
contain caffeine and all use a lot of sugar. Lucozade, the leading
brand of glucose drink, contains the yellow azo dye sunset yellow
(E110) and the preservatives sodium benzoate (E211) and sodium
metabisulphite (E223): all three of these additives have been
reported to cause allergy (see Chapter 10). Old stocks contain
tartrazine (E102). Lucozade also includes glucose syrup made from
maize (corn), cirtric acid, lactic acid, vitamin C and flavourings
which are based on lemon, orange and lime oils and a very small
amount of caffeine. Some supermarkets produce their own brand
of glucose drink with similar additives.

If you want to drink a fizzy drink, make your own with
carbonated mineral water or try 7-Up which contains carbonated
water, sugar, citric acid (E330), sodium citrate (E331) and natural
flavourings. Diet 7-Up has different ingredients.

## Tonic water

Two people said that quinine in tonic water affected them. One
asthma sufferer avoided it and one lady in her mid-fifties claimed
that when she eliminated it with white bread, her rash which took
the form of red rings disappeared: she had suffered from it on and
off since her teens.

## Milk

Cows', goats', sheep's: see Chapter 6.

# Soya milk

Soya milk is made from soya beans with some sugar and a little salt added. It has slightly more protein than cows' milk, but contains less fat, calcium and vitamins. Small children, who drink soya milk as a substitute for other milk, may require extra vitamins and calcium to counteract any deficiency: check with your community or hospital dietician. Fortified soya milk is available for babies; consult with your doctor or health visitor if you wish to change to it.

Soya milk tastes different to cows' milk but use it as you would ordinary milk: in drinks, with breakfast cereals and in cooking when it should be diluted with water by half its volume again. It is available ready to drink in 500 ml cartons (roughly a pint). It has a shelf life of six months unopened and has a date stamp showing its expiry date. Once opened, it will last up to three days if kept in a fridge.

# Wine, beer and spirits

I have not gone into these in this book as I believe you can easily do without them. Far too much alcohol is drunk as can be verified by Alcoholics Anonymous and other self-help groups. Alcohol can be dangerous, not only to your own health but to the health of others. More car accidents take place and wives and children are battered when alcohol is involved. You get a hangover if you drink too much and it is bad for your liver.

Beer is made from barley hops, wine from grapes, and spirits come from a variety of different fruits and vegetables. Most alcoholic drinks contain additives which do not have to be disclosed in the UK. Some migraine sufferers find they can drink white wine but not red. Others avoid all wines, sherry and port but can drink whisky and champagne. Abstain or at least cut down on your consumption so that if you occasionally have a glass, you will know if you get after effects from it.

Notes
1   *Nitrates*, Friends of the Earth, Spring 1982.
2   *Is Migraine Food Allergy?*, J. Egger et al, The Lancet, 15 October 1983.
3   *Asthma induced by sulphur dioxide, benzoate and tartrazine contained in orange drinks*, B.J. Freedman, Clinical Allergy, Vol. 7, p.407, 1977

# 10

# Food additives

The average Briton ate about 1·5 lb of additives in 1955 and no less than 5·4 lbs in 1984, equivalent to 22 aspirin-sized tablets every day.[1] In 1985 200,000 tonnes of additives were added to the food we eat and it is estimated that on average each person now eats about 8 to 11 lbs of additives a year, with some possibly eating much more. The use of additives has increased ten-fold in the last 30 years.[2]

Just glance along the shelves of any shop or in the store cupboards of most homes and you will see the number of food colourings, preservatives, flavourings and other additives listed on the boxes, bottles and tins. Some additives can cause allergies. Only when you, the consumer, stop buying a product containing them, will the manufacturer be prompted to change the ingredients of his product.

Some additives may be necessary to keep food fresh and prevent harmful bacteria growing. However many are added to give extra long 'shelf life' and some for only cosmetic reasons – to make the food (supposedly) look more attractive. Other additives are used as a substitute for the real thing in order to make the product cheaper.

There are about 320 listed additives allowed in food today. There are also thought to be some 6,000 flavourings. Additives are divided into categories of what they do although some chemicals perform more than one job. An example is caramel which is a colouring as well as a flavouring.

Additives are classified into the following categories: acids, acidity regulators, anti-caking agents, anti-foaming agents, antioxidants, artificial sweeteners, colours, emulsifiers, emulsifying salts, flavour enhancers, flavourings, flour improvers, gelling agents, glazing agents, preservatives, raising agents, stabilizers and thickeners. All of these except flavourings have to be further identified: either by their full chemical name or by their code number. These categories are fully described in this chapter and a complete list of additives and their code numbers is given in Appendix 2.

Detailed in this chapter are the additives which appear to give people most trouble. That is not to say that others are innocent. Like all natural foods, they should each be thought about individually. This advice is fine in theory, almost impossible in practice. It is very difficult to isolate additives in this way as they are, by their nature, always eaten with other ingredients and often with other additives. A meal made up of mainly processed convenience foods can contain up to 60 additives.[2] It could be a certain mixture of additives which creates trouble.

However your diary will tell you if you can eat a food with additives which do not affect you. This will help you assess whether a particular additive is to blame. If different foods containing the same additive crop up regularly before you get symptoms, and there is no other similarity between the foods, you have probably identified the culprit. If you can otherwise eat a food but cannot eat it if it contains any additive, you must suspect the additive.

To begin with, when assessing whether any food may be causing your allergy, I suggest you stick to as near a natural diet as possible and avoid as many additives as you can. If you feel sure that you can eat certain ones, put them on your safe list.

## Colouring

Seventy one people said that colouring added to food or drink caused them trouble. Seventeen avoided all colouring; the remainder accused yellow or orange colouring apart from three who said red colouring caused symptoms. Eighteen pinpointed tartrazine (E102) and five mentioned sunset yellow (E110); 15 others said they could not drink orange squash which contains tartrazine along with other additives (see p. 150).

Tartrazine (E102) is a yellow colouring found in many foods and made my son wheeze for four days after he ate or drank something containing it. He often got a headache with it and became sick and feverish. Pauline's daughter is also affected by this additive: 'Tartrazine is a big culprit, bringing on wheezing if drunk in squash or as a rash if taken in medicine.' Marc's mother found that whenever her son had orange squash, fish fingers (both contained tartrazine), or other highly coloured foods, his behaviour worsened. And Jennie's four year old daughter gets catarrh and severe migraine if she consumes orange and yellow artificial food colouring; she is also allergic to milk. You will have read examples of allergy to food colouring throughout this book.

There are 53 different colourings allowed by law in food, drink and drugs. See Appendix 2 for the complete list. The type of colouring used in food and drink must be disclosed on labels. Colouring used in medicines and preparations such as toothpaste, vitamin drops and cough mixtures does not need to be disclosed and rarely is. The Food Labelling Regulations do not cover these items. For more information about medicines, see Chapter 12.

**Natural food colour.** You may read these words on labels: what do they mean? Natural food colour means that the colour is taken from a natural food or a natural source which is not a food, e.g. trees or plants. Examples are annatto (E160b) taken from a South American plant and carotene (E160a) taken from carrots or other vegetables. But this description can also mean the chemically-synthesised equivalents of these colours so you cannot be sure whether the colour comes from its natural source or is made in a laboratory. I am afraid you must suspect 'natural' as well as 'artificial' colours. Annatto has been shown to cause urticaria (nettlerash) in 26 per cent of a group of chronic urticaria sufferers and 10% of another group when tested under clinical conditions.[3]

**Caramel** is the most used colouring in the food processing industry, and is also a flavouring. Made from different sugars, it goes into chocolate and sugar confectionery products as well as meat products and snack foods. There are four types of caramel. The most natural form is burnt sugar and is what its name implies: sugar heated so that it changes colour. This is used in baby foods and alcoholic drinks. The other three are caustic caramel used in spirits; ammonia caramel which is used in gravy browning and baking; and ammonium sulphite caramel used in soft drinks like cola. All four are described as caramel (E150) on labels.

**Azo dyes.** There are 11 azo dyes (see box below) plus six other artificial colourings. Tartrazine (E102), sunset yellow (E110), amaranth (E123) and ponceau (E124) are the most commonly used azo dyes in that order. Tartrazine has undergone most clinical testing: asthma, rhinitis (runny nose), different skin rashes and migraine have all been provoked by this dye. The other three colours mentioned have also produced urticaria and rhinitis under medical conditions. These four colours have been banned in Norway and Sweden except in spirits, cocktail cherries and lump

---

## Azo dyes

| Code number | Colouring |
|---|---|
| **Yellow** | |
| E102 | Tartrazine |
| 107 | Yellow 2G |
| E110 | Sunset yellow FCF, Orange yellow S |
| **Red** | |
| E122 | Carmoisine, Azorubine |
| E123 | Amaranth |
| E124 | Ponceau 4R, Cochineal red A, New cochine |
| 128 | Red 2G |
| E180 | Pigment rubine, Lithol rubine BK |
| **Black** | |
| E151 | Black PN, Brilliant black BN |
| **Brown** | |
| 154 | Brown FK |
| 155 | Chocolate brown HT, Brown HT |

A food need not be the colour of the dye as more than one colour is often used, e.g. green and red coloured foods often contain the yellow colouring tartrazine (E102).

---

fish roe (caviar). Amaranth (E123) is also banned in the USA and Israel plus France and Italy (except in caviar). Norway has, in fact, banned all azo dyes and their use is highly restricted in Sweden, Finland, Austria, Greece and Japan.[2]

Medical evidence has shown that people sensitive to aspirin may also react to azo dyes (as well as the benzoate group of preservatives). Twelve years ago in Sweden a test was carried out on eight patients with aspirin sensitivity. Seven reacted with asthma, urticaria or both after tartrazine was given to them.[4]

You may find you or your child react to one azo dye but not to the others. Think of them individually whilst discovering the cause of your allergy but remember there may be a link.

**Other artificial colourings** There are six additional artificial colourings apart from azo dyes. Sometimes called coal tar dyes, they are also considered suspect and should be eaten with caution: quinoline yellow (E104), erythrosine BS (E127), patent blue V (E131), indigo carmine (E132), brilliant blue FCF (E133) and green S, lissamine green (E142).

---

## Foods which may contain colouring

| | |
|---|---|
| Beefburgers (frozen) | Meat dishes (frozen and tinned) |
| Biscuits | Mustard |
| Breadcrumbs | Pies |
| Breakfast cereals | Pickles |
| Cakes | Puddings |
| Crisps | Relishes |
| Custard | Salad cream |
| Fish fingers and other products | Sausages |
| Fruit (tinned) | Snack foods |
| Ice cream and cones | Soups (tinned and packets) |
| Jams | Soft Drinks |
| Jellies | Vegetables (tinned) |
| Margarine | Yogurt (flavoured) |
| Marzipan | |

# Why is so much colouring added to food?

Is it necessary? Does it perform a useful function? Many reasons are given by food manufacturers for the inclusion of colouring in their products. Here are a few and judge for yourself.

**You expect an orange drink to look orange and a strawberry ice cream to look pink.** True but only because the customer has very little choice in the matter and has not been told that a paler version tastes exactly the same but does not contain colouring. Strawberry yoghurt without colouring looks almost white but can still taste delicious. Italian lemon or vanilla ice creams look white and not yellow like their English counterparts yet there can be no doubt that Italian ice creams are superb. If the labelling and advertising of a product explained that what you are buying looks different because it is colour free, the public would soon appreciate its merits and buy that product.

**We have to ensure that each batch of our products remains the same colour.** Why? Again why cannot the manufacturers state clearly that there may be a difference of colour in their product only because no colouring has been added.

**The natural colouring of some foods gets destroyed during heat processing and storage (e.g. canned vegetables and fruit) or bleached when preservatives are used, or may alter after some time.** Strong arguments you may think but still not valid if the buying public is aware of what they mean. We have got used to eating very green peas and other brightly coloured foods. If they were not that colour, would we think there was something wrong with them? Not if the label told us that they were that colour because they contained no added colouring. Food which lasts less than 18 months must have a date stamp on the packaging telling you when the food is no longer suitable to eat. If the food has a longer shelf life, you will not know how long it has been kept. This could be a valid reason for revising the law so that all packaged foods have a sell-by date no matter how long the shelf life of the product. This way the buyer would be assured that the product was still edible.

**Some foods would have no colour if none was added. Sweets, instant desserts and ice lollies for example.** If a food is worth eating, it should be eaten regardless of its colour and on its merits of goodness and taste.

**Children are attracted to brightly coloured foods.** Maybe so. But if these foods are going to cause trouble, your children would do well to avoid them. In fact the Food Additives and Contaminants Committee recommends that colouring should not be added to foods specifically prepared for babies and young children[5] and most manufacturers comply with this. However the recommendation does beg the question: if very small children should not eat these colourings, what about slightly older children or in fact any child who eats the same food as the rest of the family?

## Foods which must not be coloured

Colouring is not allowed by law to be added to raw and unprocessed meat, game, poultry, fish, fruit and vegetables.[11] Tea, coffee and milk including condensed and dried, must also be free from colouring. However meat must be health stamped with a violet dye called methyl violet – a dye not permitted for use in food itself. If you buy meat with this dye on it, cut it off before cooking. There is a chance the dye is in processed meat products as the manufacturers find it difficult to remove. Citrus fruit may also be stamped with the dye; peel it before eating and don't suck the skin.

## Flavouring

There are known to be over 3,000 natural or artificially manufactured 'nature-identical' flavourings and over 350 artificial flavourings which can be used in processed food. The Labelling Regulations allow both kinds to be labelled just 'flavouring'. This is a conservative estimate of the amount of flavourings used. Some flavourings chemists reckon the number to be nearer 6,000.[2]

Natural flavourings are taken from vegetables, fruits and nuts such as leeks, garlic, pineapple, strawberries and cashew nuts; herbs and spices, for instance dill, hollyhock, chervil; or plants which are not normally eaten like silver fir, birch or carrot seeds. Artificial flavourings are based on many chemicals and include ones related to the preservatives, benzoate and sulphur dioxide, described later in this chapter.

Just because a flavour is natural does not mean you cannot be allergic to it: it may be derived from a fruit, vegetable or nut you cannot eat or if you are allergic to a certain tree pollen, it might be the flavouring extracted from that tree which is causing the problem. Some natural flavours are extracted by means of a chemical.

Not many people mentioned flavourings as a cause of their symptoms although some did cut them out along with colourings and maybe preservatives. Dr Feingold in his diet for hyperactive children recommends them to avoid all artificial flavouring.

You will find it almost impossible to track down whether any particular flavouring is causing your allergy but if you suspect a flavouring in a product, you might ask the manufacturer what it is. If you find a brand which adds 'flavour' and you can eat it without symptoms, stick to that brand, although the flavour may be changed without you being aware of it.

## Flavour enhancers

**Monosodium glutamate** (621) is the most commonly used flavour enhancer. Twenty four people reported it made them unwell. Six suffered headaches and a solicitor from Wales gave the following description of what monosodium glutamate does to him: 'hot flushes, blinding headache, distorted vision, acute sensitivity of the eyes to light, the ears to sound and the skin to touch, periodic and very unpleasant increased heart and breathing rate and an even viler temper than usual.'

Five people suffered asthma attacks from it including Betty who wrote: 'I have suffered from hayfever turning to asthma for most of my life. A few years ago my homoeopathic doctor told me that it was possible that some ingredients were better avoided to allay allergies. I am very careful to avoid any foods which contain monosodium glutamate.'

Three people found monosodium glutamate provoked their

eczema and a further two said that it caused their face or body to swell. Anne wrote: 'About 10 years ago, my husband developed an allergy – first symptoms were swelling of hands, feet, an eye or perhaps an ear with large red weals on various parts of his body. The attacks would come at odd intervals, sometimes maybe a year would elapse without one. We never knew when it would happen. We saw four doctors and attended a skin hospital. We received no constructive help apart from being told he was "allergic to something" and being given bottles and bottles of pills and cream which did nothing. The attacks became more and more severe and his joints were becoming so stiff that at these times he could hardly walk. The swellings became more severe, his temperature would shoot up and his body felt like a furnace.' Anne's husband went to an allergy clinic, was told to throw away his pills and put on a strict diet after which foods were gradually introduced. Anne says: 'It took six weeks to pinpoint and it turned out to be monosodium glutamate; which explained why, when the attacks occurred, they were lasting so long because he was still eating the substance that was poisoning him.'

Monosodium glutamate caused three people the 'shakes', two children to become hyperactive and one lady's arthritis to get worse. One gentleman stated it was 'death to his hiatus hernia', and Hugh claimed it caused him and his wife to sleep badly with bad dreams (see p. 50).

I was gratified to receive this letter from Vivienne: 'I read with interest your published letter which gave me an insight into an allergy my daughter seems to have. It started two years ago with her having almost constant earache and sore throats (necessitating a tonsillectomy). She also threw tantrums, never slept a night through and had a permanent sore bottom.

'By pure chance I spoke to another mum with a similar problem who had taken her child off milk. I followed suit with almost miraculous results. However as time went by, it appeared I had not quite uncovered everything. So after reading your letter I took her off monosodium glutamate and I think now that was the other problem.'

You may have heard that monosodium glutamate causes the

'Chinese Restaurant Syndrome'. This is because the additive is often used in Chinese cooking, though by no means all Chinese restaurants cook with it. This is Anna's description of it: 'I was about 35 and passed out several times after a warning of less than a minute each time, with a very rapid heart beat which gave rise to an inability to breathe normally for a minute or more; when I recovered I was bathed in sweat and had slurred speech and a total lack of balance for some time. The attacks were followed by a feeling of incredible well being. After several examinations and tests it was diagnosed as Chinese Restaurant Syndrome and I learned to avoid monosodium glutamate.'

The Chinese Restaurant Syndrome was first named in 1968 by Dr Kwok, a medical researcher in America, in a letter to the New England Journal of Medicine. He described his symptoms after eating in Chinese restaurants as he did not get the same symptoms whilst eating food cooked at home. 'I have experienced a strange syndrome whenever I have eaten out in a Chinese restaurant, especially one that served Northern Chinese food. The syndrome which usually begins 15 to 20 minutes after I have eaten the first dish, lasts for about two hours, without any hangover effect. The most prominent symptoms are numbness at the back of the neck, gradually radiating to both arms and the back, general weakness and palpitation ... I had not heard of the syndrome until I received complaints of the same symptoms from Chinese friends of mine, both medical and non-medical people.' Following Dr Kwok's

| **Foods which may contain monosodium glutamate** | |
|---|---|
| Bacon | Pasta dishes (tinned) |
| Crisps | Sauce mixes |
| Frozen battered and | Salami |
|    breadcrumbed fish | Savoury snacks |
| Frozen fish in sauces | Soups (tinned and packets) |
| Gravy mixes | Stock cubes |
| Hamburgers (frozen) | Stuffing |
| Meat products (frozen | Vegetables (frozen |
|    and tinned) |    cooked in sauce) |

letter a survey in Boston showed that some 25 per cent of those responding to a questionnaire said they experienced from mild to moderately severe symptoms after eating Chinese restaurant food.

**What is monosodium glutamate?** Found naturally in seaweed, it is most frequently prepared from sugar beet. It used to be prepared from wheat gluten but no longer is. Although it does not have a prominent flavour of its own, it brings out the flavour of prepared meat, fish and some vegetable products by stimulating your taste buds. It is often used in foods containing salt as it reduces the amount of salt needed.

Also called sodium hydrogen L-glutamate, sodium glutamate and glutamic acid sodium salt, its code number is 621. Glutamic acid is found naturally in many vegetables, meat and fish but because it is released slowly into the bloodstream, it is not believed to cause the same reaction. Monopotassium glutamate (622), calcium glutamate (623) and L-glutamic acid (620) are also allowed but are not widely used.

**Children and monosodium glutamate.** Monosodium glutamate is not allowed to be used in the preparation of food specially prepared for babies and young children. However it is widely used in flavoured crisps and snacks which many children eat in large quantities. It also goes into most brands of frozen hamburgers and fishfingers. As with colourings, why should small children not eat monosodium glutamate when their slightly older brothers and sisters are encouraged to eat so much?

**Other flavour enhancers.** Manufacturers are beginning to realise that some consumers are avoiding monosodium glutamate and are substituting other flavour enhancers. Flavour enhancers should always be distinguished as such followed by the name or code number. A full list is given in Appendix 2. These like monosodium glutamate are not allowed in food specifically prepared for babies and young children.

# Preservatives

Twenty nine people said they avoided some or all preservatives in their diet. Most excluded other additives as well especially colourings and flavourings. Nine mothers of hyperactive children said their children benefited greatly from an additive-free diet.

Patricia wrote about her son who is now 13 years old: 'Daniel was a hyperactive baby. The only help I got from the medical profession was drugs to "calm him down". After reading an article in an Australian paper about additives in food, I decided to take the advice and cut out all foods with colourings and preservatives to see if there was any change in his behaviour. I cannot say there was a dramatic improvement at first but he did begin to sleep at night. By the time he started school, he could sit on a chair for more than two minutes without falling off. He is now normal in his behaviour, sleeps well and is doing very well at school.'

Six people said preservatives were one of the causes of their asthma and six said the same about their eczema. Dorothy accused all additives in foods of triggering off asthmatic attacks in her small son and another mother from Cheshire said that amongst other foods and colours, her son could not take any preservatives as they caused him outbreaks of eczema. Two people said they avoided preservatives because they caused stomach upsets and two because of migraine.

There are 35 preservatives allowed by law to go into food. These prolong the life of a food or drink, delaying the time the food takes to go off. Preservatives stop harmful bacteria and moulds growing which could make you ill. Some people say they are a means of keeping stale food edible. There are four individual groups of preservatives which you should be aware of:

**Benzoates.** There are ten benzoate preservatives: benzoic acid (E210), sodium benzoate (E211) and their derivatives E212 to E219. They are used in many squashes and fruit drinks, pickles, sauces and fruit or nut yogurts. Benzoyl peroxide is a bleaching agent, sometimes used to whiten flour, and is related to this group. Clinical tests have shown that these preservatives can cause skin complaints, asthma and rhinitis[3], and hyperactive children are advised not to eat or drink anything containing them.

**Sulphur dioxide** (E220) and its derivatives E221 to E227 are used in many foods, e.g. processed meat, drinks and fruits. One clinical test has reported sensitivity to sulphur dioxide: eight out of 14 asthmatic patients reacted to consuming sulphur dioxide[7] and there have been reports of people having breathing difficulties when inhaling it. Sodium metabisulphate (E223) may cause food aversion and skin reactions[8] as well as behaviour disturbances in children.[10]

**Nitrates and nitrites.** There are four of these preservatives: potassium nitrite (E249), sodium nitrite (E250), sodium nitrate (E251) and potassium nitrate (E252). These are used in meat products such as bacon, ham, sausages, salami and canned meats. The nitrate turns into nitrite in the meat which causes the processed meat to retain its red-pink colour. These preservatives are also allowed in some cheeses (see p. 118 for full list). Clinical tests have shown that sodium nitrite can provoke attacks of urticaria (nettlerash), stomach disorders and headaches[6] and behaviour disturbances in children.[10]

In 1978 the Food Additives and Contaminants Committee of the Ministry of Agriculture recommended that 'every effort should continue to be made to eliminate the use of nitrate and reduce nitrite levels as soon as practicable'. Food specifically prepared for babies and young children should not contain added nitrite or nitrate. If they are no good for young children, they are probably no good for the rest of us. Their use is restricted in most European countries.[2]

**Propionic acid** (E280) and its derivatives E281 to E283 are used in baked foods, bread and dairy produce. E280 has been shown to cause behaviour disturbances in children during a trial carried out in Australia[10] and may cause headaches.[8]

## Antioxidants

There are 13 antioxidants allowed in food in the UK. They are used to prevent fat and oil turning rancid. Two groups have come under some criticism.

**Gallates** Propyl gallate (E310), octyl gallate (E311) and dodecyl gallate (E312) have been reported to casue gastric irritation and problems to asthma sufferers and people sensitive to aspirin.[8] These additives are not allowed in food specifically prepared for babies and young children.

**BHA (E320) and BHT (E321).** In 1963 the Food Stadards Committee recommended that BHT (E321) no longer be permitted in food. However in the light of representations by the food industry and further research, in 1965 the permitted amounts were halved. Research into adverse effects is still being evaluated. Clinical tests have shown both these antioxidants can cause skin disorders.[3] They have also been reported to cause asthma[9]; and hyperactive children are advised not to eat anything containing them. Both these antioxidants are found in most crisps and savoury snacks and some biscuits, pastries, milk desserts and bottled sauces although paradoxically they are not permitted by law to be used in foods specifically prepared for babies and young children. Lard and other solid fats may also contain one or other of them.

## Emulsifiers and stabilizers

An emulsifier helps mix two ingredients together, e.g. eggs and oil; a stabilizer helps keep the mixture intact so that it does not separate again. Both are found in many foods including bread, cakes and pastries, ice cream, margarine, chocolate and sugar confectionery, some soft drinks and milk products. They are also used in many processed convenience foods. In the late 1950s there was an outbreak of 'Dutch margarine disease'. It took the form of a skin rash which erupted when some people consumed a particular brand of margarine. This was attributed to an emulsifier used in it.[3] Stearates 430 and 431 may also cause skin reactions.[8]

## Modified starch

Starch is found naturally in grains like maize, wheat, potato, tapioca and sago. Modified starch can be made from any of these starches and has been treated in some way, usually with chemicals.

These include arsenic, lead, copper, zinc and sulphur dioxide. Modified starch is used extensively in the food processing industry. It acts as a thickener, for instance in sauces, chocolates and sweets; it helps prevent caking in foods such as icing sugar; and it stabilises foods like salad dressing where the fat or oil are likely to separate. Ordinary starch will not stand up to many processing procedures: that is why it is chemically modified.

## Enzymes

Enzymes are found naturally in all foods. They are also present in your own body to aid digestion of food. Enzymes cause chemical changes to take place. Natural enzymes derived from animal or plant tissue, are rennet, pepsin, trypsin, papain and bromelain but very few natural enzymes are used in food. They are usually chemically synthesised. They are used in the production of bread, biscuits, cheesemaking and brewing. Their use is not disclosed on labelling.

## Artificial sweeteners

**Saccharin** is the most widely used artificial sweetener; as a tablet, powder or liquid, it is added to drinks and food to sweeten them without the need to add extra calories. It is also used in many processed foods and drinks and must appear on labelling.

Four people in my survey said they avoided saccharin. One lady suffered from asthma. Another said she had suffered from boils for the past 18 years. After regular visits to her doctor for penicillin and hospital visits when nothing was discovered, she began to think about when it had all started and tied it down to the taking of saccharin. 'I decided to stop taking anything which had saccharin in it and I am delighted to tell you I have not had a boil for three years now.'

Anne wrote that she noticed a change in her small daughter after she started to drink a blackcurrant cordial with saccharin in it. 'The effect was dramatic, my daughter aged three, suffered terrible nightmares and bedwetting on a totally bewildering scale. After two disrupted nights, I thought of all possible causes. It seemed to point to the change of drink and the introduction of saccharin to her diet. This was a correct assumption and after 48 hours all was normal again. This problem of saccharin is also shared by another friend whose daughter also developed nightmares and bedwetting from drinking lemonade.'

The fourth letter came from a lady who said her husband became very 'twitchy' from it. 'Whilst sitting down in the evening, his legs would twitch constantly and he would have to get up and move about. By elimination we worked this out to be saccharin.'

Saccharin has come under a lot of criticism in recent years because it was shown to cause cancer in rats when fed very large doses. Although some medical opinion says these tests were unrealistic as humans do not consume such large amounts and what affects rats may not affect humans in the same way, the results were sufficiently frightening for the authorities to ban the use of saccharin in Canada. In the USA a warning is now printed on all food containing it saying: 'Use of this product may be hazardous to your health. This product contains saccharin which has been determined to cause cancer in laboratory animals.'

**Other sweeteners.** Recently a number of other artificial sweeteners have been allowed. A full list is given in Appendix 2.

## More additives

Other groups (categories) of additives which you will come across are described below together with the functions they perform. They should be followed by the name of the actual additive used or its code number on food labels.

**Acids** provide a tart flavour and have a preservative effect. They also aid the release of carbon dioxide when present in raising agents.

**Acidity regulators/buffers** change or maintain the acidity or alkalinity levels in food. They aid preservation, add or alter flavour or tartness and assist in texture development, colour retention and the action of raising agents.

**Anti-caking agents** prevent the 'caking' or lumping of finely powdered substances such as salt.

**Anti-foaming agents** prevent liquids boiling over and reduce scum forming by breaking down foams.

**Bleaching agents** bleach or whiten flour and bread. See White flour p. 123.

**Bulking agents** add bulk to food without adding extra calories. They are primarily intended for slimming foods. As they are not usually digested, they act as a source of fibre.

**Diluents** dilute or dissolve other additives, often colours.

**Firming agents** help maintain the firmness or crispness of foods such as fruit and vegetables which may soften and fall apart in extreme conditions such as canning or freezing.

**Flour improvers** extend the elastic properties and aid the development of dough in bread making. See Flour on p. 123.

**Freezants** extract heat from food which is consequently frozen by direct contact.

**Glazing agents** produce a sheen on the surface of, for example, sweets and dried fruit. They also provide a protective coating in some cases.

**Humectants** retain moisture when added to food preventing it from rapidly becoming dry due to the evaporation of its water content. They may be added to confectionery.

**Propellants** are gases or volatile liquids used to expel foods from aerosol containers e.g. whipped cream.

**Raising agents** promote aeration creating a lighter texture and increased volume when used in baked products.

**Release agents** prevent foods from sticking to other surfaces with which they come in contact during manufacture or packaging.

**Thickening or gelling agents** form gels which modify the texture and create stability in certain foods. They are usually made of starch or gum but the latter is more expensive and therefore less widely used.

## Notes

1  *Food Additives*, Ecoropa Information Sheet 12, 1984.
2  *A Report on Food Additives*, Melanie Miller, The London Food Commission, October 1985.
3  EEC Reports of the Scientific Committee for Food (twelfth series) 1982 EUR 7823 sold in the UK by HMSO.
4  *Urticaria and asthma induced by food and drug additives in patients with aspirin hypersensitivity*, Juhlin, Michaelsson and Zefferstrom, Journal of Allergy and Clinical Immunology, 1972.
5  Interim Report on the Review of the Colouring Matter in Food Regulations, 1973.
6  *Clinical Reactions to Food* edited by M. H. Lessof, John Wiley & Sons, 1983.
7  *Asthma induced by sulphur dioxide, benzoate and tartrazine contained in orange drinks*, B. J. Freedman, Clinical Allergy, 1977.
8  *E for Additives*, Maurice Hanssen, Thorsons Publishers, 1984.
9  *The Right Way to Eat,* Miriam Polunin, J. M. Dent & Sons Ltd, 1984.
10  *Salicylates, oligoantigenic diets, and behaviour,* Anne Swain et al, The Lancet, 6 July 1985.
11  But it may still occur if added to animal or fish feed or is injected into orange trees according to *Food Additives*, Erik Millstone, Penguin Special, 1986.

# 11

# Eating out

What should you do when you want to eat out? Perhaps you are invited to friends or want to go for a meal in a pub or restaurant. What should you do when you take a holiday or travel abroad? Food in hospital can also be a problem. Here are a few tips.

## Visiting friends

Do not feel you have to be a recluse eating only in your own home. If you get an invitation to eat a meal at a friend's house, accept it with pleasure. If there is anything you cannot eat, tell your hostess in advance. Indicate what you can eat; it will make her plans much easier. At the table, do not be afraid to refuse food which you know will disagree with you. Explain your situation tactfully and you will only get sympathy. Ask your hostess what ingredients went into the food: often a topic of conversation in any event. Note them down in your diary later. Not only will you be able to check whether the ingredients were all right for you to eat; you may also get a useful recipe. For advice on children visiting friends, see 'A child's diaries' on p.62.

## School meals

If your child is allergic to any food or you think he or she may be, take my advice and send your child to school with a packed lunch. Hot meals are not better than cold ones. Sandwiches and home-made food can easily be packed and a vacuum flask containing a cold drink (like fruit juice) or a hot home-made soup can be added. You will then know exactly what your child is eating (unless he picks at someone else's food at lunch or during break).

## Pub grub

Go for plain food. Read the labels on crisps and nuts bought in packets. Do not eat them if they are already served in bowls on the counter; they may contain something (a flavour enhancer or colouring) which can disagree with you. A ploughman's lunch consisting of bread, cheddar cheese and tomato will be okay if you can eat these ingredients: alternatively, choose a salad and check if any dressing is added and what it contains. Watch out for pies and hot dishes which may include many hidden ingredients. Ask if the fried chicken or fish and chips in the basket is made from fresh ingredients or (more likely) arrives on the premises frozen and only needs reheating: frozen foods contain many additives including colouring (catering packs now contain a list of ingredients so it should be possible to check).

## Restaurants

Restaurants vary widely in the choice and quality of the food they provide. Many serve only precooked, frozen meals: all the chef has to do is pop the food into a micro-wave oven to heat it up. Many of these dishes will contain additives which their fresh counterparts do not require. But even freshly cooked food needs to be considered carefully as sauces, seasonings and tasty-sounding concoctions may well contain hidden ingredients you would wish to avoid.

Your only way of solving this problem is to get the waiter to ask the chef what ingredients go into a particular dish and point out what might be harmful to you. Unfortunately even the person in the kitchen might not know. Does the home-made soup include a stock cube containing a flavour enhancer or has any milk, cream, wheat thickener or egg been added? Does the ice cream in the pudding contain colouring? Are there certain vegetables, meats or grains in the stew you should avoid? Are the vegetables fresh, frozen or, heaven preserve us, tinned. Go for plain food: steak (but check what the seasoning consists of) or chops, fish (the same applies), fresh vegetables and fruit. If you find you can eat the food, you have probably discovered your favourite restaurant. But remember ingredients can change from time to time. Chinese restaurants are famous for adding monosodium glutamate (621) and I have discovered that tartrazine (E102) and ponceau 4R (E124), two colourings, are added to Tandoori recipes in most Indian restaurants.

## Hamburger restaurants

If you want a quick meal and can eat beef and white rolls, hamburgers might make a suitable snack. McDonald's, Burger King and Wendy hamburgers are made only of beef: nothing is added before cooking. Wendy and McDonald's add plain salt as the burger is cooking, Burger King adds nothing. Wimpy hamburgers contain added beef fat and seasoning of salt, spice extracts and the flavour enhancer monosodium glutamate (621). Check with your local hamburger restaurant what ingredients go into its hamburgers, and while ordering, ask the chef or waiter not to use any seasoning unless you can check what it is.

Avoid any relishes or pickles which might affect you. If you cannot check the ingredients, ask the waiter or chef to exclude these from your order. Milk shakes and other soft drinks should also be avoided if the equivalent cannot be drunk at home. Colouring is bound to be added to milk shakes and ice cream.

## Pizza parlours

Pizzas are mostly prepared fresh on the premises. The dough is made from flour, water, vegetable oil, salt and sugar. A tomato sauce is then spread over it. The recipe for this is usually fresh tomatoes, salt, tomato puree and oregano (a herb). Mozarella or a mixture of cheddar and mozarella cheese is sprinkled on top. Other ingredients may be added such as salami, mushrooms, peppers, olives or onions according to your order.

Think of all these ingredients separately if you wish to buy a pizza and also check that no other seasoning, additives or ingredients have also gone into the recipe which may disagree with you. I have found that most pizzas are okay for my son but occasionally a pizza from a newly tried restaurant, even in Italy, has come under suspicion. I could not check the exact ingredients so I cannot be sure whether there was anything else in the pizza which made him ill.

If you order a salad with your pizza, check whether the vegetables are acceptable and enquire what the salad dressing is made of.

## Fish and chips

As most fish and chips are deep fried in the restaurant, especially take-away establishments, ask the fryer what the batter and oil are made of: he should know. Check if the potatoes have been frozen and what the pickles consist of.

## Fried chicken and other fast food take-aways

The producers of Kentucky Fried Chicken will not reveal the ingredients they use so avoid their food. If you can check what ingredients go into other fast foods, then they may be acceptable to you: but be careful.

## Take-away sandwich bars

Choose sandwiches with plain, readily-identifiable ingredients. Ask whether butter or margarine is used. Watch out for sauces and relishes which may contain hidden ingredients. Ask the sandwich bar man about the ingredients he uses. As he probably makes up the sandwiches, he will know what goes into them. Don't start asking him questions at his busiest time when there is a long queue: you won't get the answers you are looking for!

Make a mental note of the sandwiches you can eat (and record them in your diary) but remember ingredients do change from time to time. Chicken, for instance, may be roasted in the shop or it may come processed without bones: according to my husband, the processed meat tastes disgusting and contains many additives. The same can apply to turkey and some other meats.

## Travelling abroad

You should have no fear of going on holiday abroad, even if you have a food allergy, though if you don't speak the language you will find it more difficult to enquire about ingredients in restaurants and identify ingredients on labels. Most countries have labelling laws similar to the UK – and in some countries, notably USA, France and Italy, you may find it easier to obtain additive-free foods than at home. Countries within the European Community and some others use the same coding for additives as the UK.

In general you would be sensible to select a holiday destination where you can choose what you eat. A self-catering apartment or cottage gives you the option of full control over what you or your child eats. If you try a newly discovered food for the first time, remember to note it down in your diary: it will need to pass your 'safe' food test.

**Air journeys.** Meals on planes come pre-packed in plastic containers: starters and main courses arrive unnamed and it will be impossible to discover what the ingredients are as the preparers of the food will be many hours and miles away when you eat the meal. If you want to be on the safe side, take your own food with you.

Packets of condiments and sauces usually disclose their ingredients as do some desserts but the amount of chemicals added to one chocolate pudding served on a flight should put off the heartiest appetite. Although described as 'new improved', it contained no less than 11 different additives. The ingredients in tiny print ran right round the container lid.

Watch out for similar foods in similar packets containing different ingredients. When I took a trip on one airline packets of peanuts were given out with drinks. One packet prepared in New York contained peanuts roasted in vegetable oil and salt; another identical looking packet contained peanuts, salt, starch, monosodium glutamate, edible gum and spices – it was packed in the Isle of Man.

**France.** The French really care about food and eating out is a national pastime. Shop food is labelled under laws similar to those in the UK though colouring is not used nearly so extensively as in Britain. One packet of ham carried the information: 'This product is pale because it is not artificially coloured'. You are less likely to encounter pre-prepared food in a French restaurant. But don't assume everything is home-made. For instance gherkins served at the table in an old-fashioned pickling jar may have been lifted out of a catering pack five minutes beforehand and could contain colouring and preservative. If you are not sure, ask but be prepared for outrage at the suggestion that anything is not 'à la maison'.

**Spain.** Most people who go to Spain go on package holidays including full or half board. That means mass catering and the same sort of problems your children will experience with school food. Many hotels are self-service so you are unlikely to be able to get a waiter or waitress to enquire about ingredients on your behalf. If you want to enjoy a holiday in Spain, try self-catering.

**USA.** If you take a holiday in Northern America and self-cater, you will find that the contents of packaged, canned and bottled foods are labelled in much the same way as their British counterparts. Colouring is not identified individually except for tartrazine coded FD&C Yellow No. 5. Some ingredients of ingredients may be disclosed, e.g. shortening contains hydrogenised soyabean oil and/or hydrogenated palm oil and/or beef fat but others may not: tinned tuna fish in vegetable broth does not disclose on its label which vegetable is used and what else it contains; and a bottle of salad dressing described as made with only natural ingredients uses pickle which was not more adequately described (most bottled pickles in the USA contain additives).

Although Americans seem more aware than the British of the marketability of 'natural' foods, beware of misleading claims. I have seen a packet of crisps proclaiming no preservatives but containing colouring and the flavour enhancer monosodium glutamate; natural flavoured ice cream may contain artificial colouring. Study labels carefully before you buy or eat a product.

Eating out must be undertaken with caution. Asking whether hamburgers or waffles (a type of pancake) are made on the premises is not sufficient. Flavouring containing the flavour enhancer monosodium glutamate, known as MSG in the USA, or other additives may be used with the fresh minced meat which makes a hamburger; waffles may come from a packet of mix containing ingredients other than flour and egg. Waiters and waitresses however seem to understand what you mean when you say you or your child is allergic to certain foods or ingredients and are usually very helpful. They will check with the cook whether a meal on the menu contains any ingredient which disagrees with you and the cook may even prepare the food omitting the allergy causing ingredient or ingredients.

**Italy.** Perhaps it is because Italians care so much about their health and their children that they label their food so effectively. Glance at any Italian magazine and you will see many food advertisements proclaiming their product's natural ingredients. 'Senza colorante' (without colouring), 'ingredienti naturali' (natural ingredients) feature in many advertisements and appear prominently on labels. Food labelling on packaged foods gives a full list of ingredients indicating all additives by their codes, which are the same as in England.

Eating out in Italy is a pleasure. Most food is prepared fresh on the premises and the use of local produce including many different herbs makes Italian cooking one of the most delicious in the world. Restaurants and trattorias are often small family affairs. Mention to the waiter that you or your child is 'allergiche' and the chef will often appear from the kitchen to explain exactly what he has put into the making of a particular dish. You do not need to understand all he says. Learn the name of the foods or additives that you are allergic to and you will be told what dishes to avoid.

Ice cream (gelato) which originates from Italy and tastes completely different from its English factory-produced counterpart, is frequently made on the premises and in some parts of the country a notice nearby discloses its ingredients. Lemon ice cream must not be coloured by law. Ask for it to be scooped out into little containers which come with a spoon as cones may contain other ingredients and additives you wish to avoid.

## Hospitals

Hospital, where you go to get better, is often the place least likely to achieve this where food allergy is concerned. Although the choice of meals has increased and the food is nutritionally better than in the past, meals within hospitals still vary tremendously.

Often you will find it very difficult to identify ingredients used in dishes which arrive on your tray despite the fact that you have ordered them yourself. Enlist the help of the hospital dietician, who may be able to sort out suitable meals for you. A choice of salads, wholemeal bread and plain foods like boiled eggs, cheese or fish is often available but meat may well come covered in gravy or seasoned in some way and vegetables may be tinned. The use of a fridge may be made available to you where you can keep food brought in by friends and relatives and of course fruit, your favourite breakfast cereal, biscuits and even vegetables can be left by your bedside.

Watch out for drugs which are coloured or may contain anything else you are allergic to. You may have to stand up to some strong argument from doctors and nurses but ask for equivalents without these. Unfortunately you are at your most vulnerable in hospital, both physically and intellectually. The fact that even adults become child-like creatures in hospital is undisputed by almost all patients I have met. To argue or even voice an opinion with 'someone in authority' can be trying, upsetting and frustrating. Nevertheless stand up for your rights as you see them.

# 12

# Medicines

It is unfortunate, if not outrageous, that the laws which enable the consumer to know which ingredients and additives go into the food and drink he buys do not cover the medicines and other pharmaceutical preparations he uses. Both prescription and non-prescription medicines and preparations which range from painkillers, cough mixtures and lozenges to vitamin pills and toothpaste contain many ingredients besides the 'active' drug itself. Only the active ingredients need be described; all the other ingredients and additives are rarely, if ever, disclosed.

## Active ingredients

Some people are allergic to the active ingredient itself, for instance penicillin or aspirin. Paracetamol is an alternative painkiller to aspirin. Barbiturates, as a sedative or tranquillizer, can also cause trouble. Mary writes: 'I am allergic to a barbiturate. I come out in red, raised spots, like measles, and long red weals on the skin, following nerve lines. I have never taken barbiturates until I was given them whilst pregnant with my son to help me sleep towards the end of my pregnancy. The reaction was almost immediate, after taking just two of the pills.'

Doctors are on the look-out for known side-effects caused by the active ingredient of a drug and may tell you about them; if your doctor does not, ask. Occasionally, a warning may be issued in a leaflet with the medicine indicating any contra-indications (side-effects) you might get. This warning only concerns the active ingredient; it will not tell you about possible allergic reactions to any of the 'inactive' ingredients.

Watch out for medicines with instructions printed on the package which may be hidden under the chemist's own label, for instance some drugs must be kept cool to retain their potency and this warning may be hidden from view.

Evidence is now being accumulated that the active ingredient of a drug can have differing effects on people because it is metabolised at different rates.[1] So what may be an acceptable dose to one person may be an overdose to another. This is rarely taken into consideration when drugs are prescribed to adults except when you end up on an operating table in hospital: the amount of anaesthetic you receive does depend on your size and weight.

Drugs can affect you in ways you don't want them to. I know of two people who were made high and excitable on a tranquilliser and one doctor believes that the oral contraceptive pill is responsible for an increase in migraine headaches, depressive mood changes and suicide attempts, allergies to food and chemicals, and cervical and breast cancer. She also believes that women taking the pill are more likely to have abnormal or allergic children.[2] Both tranquillizers and the contraceptive pill contain other ingredients and no one has researched whether any adverse symptoms are caused by them as opposed to the active ingredient.

Non-prescription drugs may also cause trouble. Phyllis suffered from chilblains so she bought 100 tablets of Pernivit over the counter at her chemist shop. The label said the adult dose was one to three tablets three times a day. She took one and within five minutes, she had a red burning rash all over her body which lasted half an hour. There was a warning printed on the bottle telling her: 'Discontinue immediately if rash appears'. Needless to say, she stopped taking them.

Do not assume that so called natural drugs sold without prescription are harmless. Mistletoe, liquorice and ginseng have been reported in the press[3] as possibly causing unpleasant side-effects.

Alternatively drugs may have no effect at all. In a recent survey,[4] over three-quarters (78 per cent) of the people who were prescribed tranquillizers for allergic symptoms reported no improvement.

# Inactive ingredients

The so-called 'inactive' ingredients include bulking and binding agents such as lactose powder (made from milk), starch (made from wheat or corn), colouring (including E102, E110 and E123), flavouring and preservatives (E200, E202, and E220). Sugar and artificial sweeteners are frequently used as well as gums and waxes, magnesium stearate (572), talc (553b), silicon dioxide (551), glycerol (E422), polyvinyl-pyrrolidone (a binder in slow release capsules) and cellulose (460-466).[5] No one except the manufacturer will know which of these are used. Your doctor and pharmacist will, almost certainly, be as ignorant as you are.

If you want to avoid a certain ingredient or additive, or want to find out what goes into the drug you are prescribed, you will run into severe difficulties. Drug companies do not usually release information about their products to members of the public. I was told that this is written into the pharmaceutical industry's code of practice which states: 'Requests from individual members of the public for information or advice on personal medical matters must always be refused and the enquirer recommended to consult his or her own doctor'.

If you are given this excuse by a drug company for not disclosing its ingredients, you will have to ask your doctor or chemist. As they will not know, they must write to or telephone the manufacturer involved. Your doctor, probably an extremely busy man or woman, might not be very eager to do this – it takes time and can mean delay especially if more than one company has to be contacted. Some hospitals have an information service which gives this sort of advice. However drug contents do change and the information might not be up to date.

Despite this, some drug companies will give you some information and I suggest you do contact them direct. If you ask them a specific question such as does the drug contain lactose, starch or a specific colouring, you will probably get an answer. Do not be afraid to contact the company: if enough people show they are concerned about what goes into a drug, then there may be a change in this ridiculous loophole in the law which prevents the consumer automatically knowing what goes into a medicine.

Due to the possibility of allergic reactions to inactive ingredients, at the beginning of 1984 the Pharmaceutical Society wrote to the Department of Health asking that disclosure of all ingredients of medicinal products should be made either on a label or as a package insert and, when appropriate, on a data sheet. This prompted the Department of Health to have informal consultations with doctors and dentists amongst others. The next stage is for the Department of Health to send out formal proposals to be discussed with interested parties. No date has been set for this so it will take several years, if at all, before labelling inactive ingredients on medicines will come about.

## Colouring in drugs

Colouring used in drugs seems to be a common reason why drugs may do more harm than good. I received several letters complaining of this. One little boy became hyperactive when prescribed Actifed syrup for his cold. It was coloured with tartrazine (E102). His mother writes: 'The return of his previous bad behaviour was most marked and convinced both my husband and myself that we were correct in our belief that food colouring reacted badly with him. We raised the subject with our GP who admitted to being sceptical but referred us to a paediatrician who agreed with our findings.'

Tartrazine (E102) was also the reason for Kathleen's added discomfort: 'After a torn back muscle, I was prescribed Equagesic (a painkiller) which I took three times a day for two days when my face swelled up alarmingly. I left the tablets off and after 24 hours the swellings subsided. However I continued to be so afflicted at intervals, sometimes once a fortnight, sometimes as often as three times a week for the next nine months.

'My doctor gave me antihistamine and talked of stress. My dentist however who saw me during one of my swellings referred me to the dental clinic where I was eventually transferred to a local dermatologist (skin doctor) who has made allergies his special interest. He quickly established the cause: tartrazine in my pain killing tablets, and after talking me through the most recent attacks, handed me a sheet of foods to be avoided. I now know that all food colourings trigger my attacks.'

Common Market scientists have recommended that 'tartrazine (or any colouring agent similarly able to provoke adverse reactions) should be removed from the formulation of any drug likely to be prescribed to allergic subjects[6].' Although colouring and other additives are voluntarily excluded from foods specifically made for babies and small children, this does not apply to drugs prescribed for them. Many children's antibiotics are coloured although non-coloured versions do exist. Pills and syrups specifically prescribed for allergic symptoms may also be coloured although pharmaceutical companies are beginning to produce colourless ones. Ask your doctor for them. In fact if you are concerned about the colour of any drug you are taking, ask if there is a non-coloured alternative.

The argument for colouring drugs is strong. Different colours make the product distinctive, both to the user and the chemist who dispenses it. There is less chance of taking the wrong pill. However there must be an alternative way of identifying pills and syrups which does not entail the use of added colour.

Some doctors say that coloured medicines have a strong psychological effect. Blue pills, for instance, make good sleeping pills and one doctor told me some patients say white ones don't work so well. In the same way, white pills are said to soothe stomach upsets in a way red ones cannot and red colouring must be used in iron tablets to encourage the thought that they strengthen the blood.

Vitamin C tablets are usually coloured orange to represent the fruit they are believed to come from. They also often contain a lot of sugar. Karin wrote about Vitamin C pills: 'Both my teenage children have suffered all their lives from allergies. I used to believe they had continual colds and gave them double doses of Haliborange tablets for extra Vitamin C. I have only recently discovered that these tablets contain the colouring tartrazine and therefore I was only adding fuel to fire their colds.'

The manufacturer of Haliborange points out that only the recommended dose should be taken as the tablets also contain Vitamins A and D (where overdoses can be dangerous). In 1983 the colouring of Haliborange was changed from tartrazine (E102) to beta-carotene (E160a). The new pack design depicts a halved orange but unhelpfully it still does not state which colouring or other additives are used. Old packs using tartrazine may still be available in some shops.

Many other non-prescription preparations including cough mixtures, sweets and lozenges are coloured, often with tartrazine and other azo dyes (see p. 158). Karin continues in her letter: 'Dental disclosing tablets can cause both my children to have tonsillitis, sore throats, raging temperatures, rashes and runny noses.' She says mouth washes and strongly coloured and flavoured toothpastes also affect them.

Mike found that the red dye used on his son's teeth made him wheeze: 'A recent visit to the dentist for fluoride treatment was illuminating. Our eldest boy aged 11 went first and had his teeth rinsed with a red dye to show up plaque areas. Within half an hour he was asthmatic and distressed. We went back to the dentist and were shown that the dye used contained tartrazine. He has since changed it and been very interested in this obvious test case which clearly demonstrated cause and response.'

Other pink dyes used for disclosing plaque may be coloured with erythrosine (E127). So also may pink mouthwashes – at the dentist as for plain water to rinse with instead. Salt water is an effective alternative to a coloured mouthwash. Fluoride supplements for children are usually artificially coloured and flavoured.

## Toothpaste

Toothpaste is made from a number of ingredients but hardly any are named on the labels of the leading brands except for the active ingredient such as fluoride. The undisclosed ingredients consist of an abrasive powder which acts as a polishing agent, a humectant to keep the toothpaste moist and which gives it that elasticity which enables you to squeeze it out of its tube, a binding agent which holds the paste intact (usually cellulose made from wood pulp), a foaming agent to make it go frothy when in your mouth, water, flavourings, all the major brands include saccharin, and often colours and a preservative.

Colgate-Palmolive manufactures Colgate Dental Cream Great Regular Flavour (the white version), Colgate Blue Minty Gel and Ultrabrite. All three use glycerine (a by-product of beef fat and nut oils) as the humectant, cellulose as the binding agent and sodium lauryl sulphate as the foaming agent. Peppermint, spearmint 'and a wealth of other flavourings' are added. Colgate Blue Minty Gel uses the preservative sodium benzoate (E211) as a flavour enhancer, brilliant blue FCF (133), an artificial colour, and titanium dioxide (E171) as colourings, and silica as its polishing agent. Colgate Dental Cream Great Regular Flavour and Ultrabrite contain no colours or preservatives and use calcium phosphate and calcium carbonate respectively as their polishing agents.

Elida Gibbs which makes Mentadent, Signal and Gibbs SR uses alumina (a mineral containing aluminium) as its polishing agent, sorbitol (E420) made from maize (corn) as its humectant, cellulose as its binding agent, sodium lauryl sulphate as its foaming agent and formalin derived from formaldehyde as its preservative (there is no formalin in Mentadent). Flavourings are many. Elida Gibbs says: 'Flavours are created by the subtle blending of a number of flavour ingredients of which there are thousands. Methol, eucalyptus, vanilla and aniseed are used but the most common ones are peppermint and spearmint.' The colour used in their white toothpaste Gibbs SR is titanium dixoide (E171); a red colour called rouge covalac (EEC Red No. 23), which is not allowed in food, was used in Signal and Mentadent when this book went to press.

Beecham Products, which produces three versions of Macleans toothpaste as well as Aquafresh, all with calcium carbonate as a polishing agent, will not disclose any other ingredients of its toothpastes except for calcium glycerophosphate which appears on labels. Certain people may be sensitive to the level of formaldehyde which goes into the Macleans Sensitive Teeth formula: their mouths may become sore but there is a warning on the label.

Proctor & Gamble which makes Crest will also not disclose the ingredients of its toothpaste but uses silica (E551) as its polishing agent.

If you suspect any ingredient in your toothpaste may contribute to your allergy, let the manufacturer know and change your brand. Go for white toothpastes – they may cause less trouble.

Alternatively use toothpastes sold in health food shops which disclose their ingredients. Unfortunately they are expensive and some children refuse to use them as they do not like the taste. The ingredients of toothpastes change from time to time so if you suspect this may have happened, check with the manufacturer.

**Notes**
1  *How drugs can turn to poison*, The Sunday Times, 2 October 1983.
2  *The contraceptive pill: its relation to allergy and illness.* Dr Ellen C. G. Grant, Journal of the Irish Allergy Treatment and Research Association, September 1983.
3  *Daily Mail*, 24 October 1983.
4  Survey on the health care of allergy sufferers, Surrey University Computer Programme, July 1983.
5  Information supplied by Bio-Health Ltd.
6  EEC Reports of the Scientific Committee for Food (Twelfth series) 1982 EUR 7823 sold in the UK by HMSO.

# 13

# Nutritional information

## Carbohydrates

Bread, breakfast cereals, potatoes and rice are good sources of carbohydrates as they also contain protein, minerals and vitamins. Jam and sugar are not good sources as apart from providing energy, they contain little else and can cause tooth decay.

## Fats

Butter, margarine, vegetable oils, milk and cheese all contain a lot of fat. So do nuts and even lean meat and some oily fish like herring and mackerel. Doctors say we eat too much fat and recommend that we cut our consumption by 20 per cent.[1] If you want to do this, grill meat and fish instead of frying, cut off fat from meat and spread your butter and margarine thinner.

## Proteins

Proteins are essential to your health as they help you grow and repair your body. If you do not eat enough carbohydrates and fat, proteins are used to provide energy instead. It is therefore important, especially for children, to eat enough carbohydrates and fats so that the protein eaten is used for its main purpose and is not just used to create heat and energy.

About two-thirds of the protein eaten in the UK comes from meat, fish, eggs and milk products. Wheat, maize and rice are also good sources and are the main providers of protein in many parts of the world. Peas, beans and nuts contain useful quantities but other root, green and leafy vegetables contain only small amounts.

## Vitamins

These are also essential to keep you healthy.

**Vitamin A (retinol)** is found in meat and fish or can be obtained from deep yellow or orange 'carotenes' found in some vegetables and fruit. Good sources are liver, kidneys, green vegetables (especially spinach), orange-yellow fruit and vegetables (especially carrots), eggs, cheese, butter, margarine, milk and fatty fish, e.g. mackerel and herring.

**B Vitamins** are not stored for long in the body so need to be constantly eaten. Substantial amounts can be lost through cooking. There are eight different B vitamins. These are listed below with the foods from which they can be adequately obtained; many of these foods contain most of them.

$B_1$ **(thiamin):** meat (especially pork, liver and kidneys), breakfast cereals, milk, bread, nuts, peas and beans.

$B_2$ **(riboflavin):** meat (especially liver), eggs, breakfast cereal, milk, cheese and almonds. Food additive numbers: E101, 101a.

$B_3$ **(nicotinic acid, niacin):** Liver, kidneys, poultry, fish, meat, breakfast cereals (with it added), wholemeal bread. Food additive number: 375.

$B_5$ **(pantothenic acid):** widespread in foods.

$B_6$ **(pyridoxine):** meat, fish, breakfast cereals, bananas.

$B_{12}$ **(cobalamin):** only in meat, fish and milk products.

**Folic acid (folate):** liver, raw green leafy vegetables, peanuts, avocado pears, oranges.

**Biotin:** Liver, kidneys, egg yolk, milk.

**Vitamin C (ascorbic acid)** should be eaten every day as it cannot be stored in the body. Substantial amounts can be lost through cooking and exposure to light and air. Good sources are blackcurrants, strawberries, kiwi fruit, grapefruit, oranges, potatoes, fresh green vegetables, tomatoes, and red and green peppers. Food additive numbers: E300 to E302.

**Vitamin D** does not usually need to be eaten as you should get enough from the sun's rays on your exposed skin. People who might not get enough this way are children, pregnant and breast-feeding mothers and dark skinned people. Good sources are fatty (oily) fish, eggs and butter (margarine has it added by law).

**Vitamin E** is found in most foods. Good sources are vegetable oils, nuts, eggs and green leafy vegetables. Food additive numbers: E306 to E309.

**Vitamin K** is in most foods and your body can make its own. Good sources are spinach, cabbage, cauliflower, peas and cereals.

## Vitamin pills

Which? magazine in a report on vitamins said: 'Do not waste your money. You should get all the vitamins you need from the food you eat.'[2] The Health Education Council agrees: 'A varied diet with plenty of fresh fruit, vegetables and cereals along with some fish, eggs, meat and dairy products will contain more than enough of all the vitamins. Unless you have a special medical reason, it is a waste of time and money to take vitamin pills.'[3]

However cutting out foods to which you think you are allergic may mean you are not getting enough vitamins in your diet and taking drugs to relieve your allergy, e.g. aspirin, antibiotics, may interfere with your body's ability to absorb vitamins. If you feel you or your child are not getting enough vitamins, ask your doctor to refer you to a hospital or community dietician or do your own research.[4]Overdoses of vitamins A, $B_6$, and D can be dangerous. Many vitamin and mineral pills are coloured and may contain other ingredients and additives to which you are allergic. Additive-free vitamin pills are available.[5]

## Minerals

The eight major minerals which keep you healthy are: calcium, phosphorus, magnesium, sodium, chlorine, potassium, iron and sulphur. You also need in smaller amounts: fluorine, zinc, copper, iodine, manganese, chromium and cobalt. All these minerals are found in most natural every day foods but are greatly reduced in processed and refined foods. Stick to natural and unrefined foods and you should not become deficient in them but take note of the following:

**Calcium** is essential for your bones, teeth and muscles. Sources of calcium are milk, cheese, white bread, hard water, bones of canned fish, watercress and cabbage. To absorb calcium you need Vitamin D.

**Iron** fortifies your blood. Usually only women of child-bearing age suffer from any deficiency. Good sources are liver, kidneys, meat, bread and breakfast cereals (if it has been added,) shellfish and spinach. Vitamin C helps absorb iron so eat plenty of fruit and vegetables.

**Sodium chloride** is salt (see p. 138).

# Fibre

Fibre is the roughage in your diet which helps food pass smoothly through your system and helps avoid constipation. It is thought to be the most important ingredient possibly lacking in most people's diet. This is because the main foods eaten are meat, eggs, dairy products and refined foods which contain none.

Good sources are bread (wholemeal contains three times as much as white), potatoes, vegetables and fruit. Bran (wheat, rice or soya bean) is also good although too much may reduce the absorption of certain minerals, e.g. calcium, zinc and iron.[6]

**Notes**
1 *Obesity,* a report by the Royal College of Physicians, 1983.
2 *Which? Magazine,* Consumers Association, January 1984
3 *Looking After Yourself,* Health Education Council, 1979.
4 For example use *The Dictionary of Vitamins,* Leonard Mervyn BSc, Thorsons Publishers Ltd, or *The Vitamin Bible,* Earl Mindell, Arlington Books.
5 From Bio-Health Ltd for example, see Appendix 1 for address.
6 *Bran does not equal fibre* by Elisabeth Morse, Self-Health Magazine, March 1984.

# Appendix 1

## Useful Addresses

**Action Against Allergy**
43 The Downs, London SW20 8HG.
Tel: 01-947 5082. Sells books about
allergy and gives information about
alternative food, relevant products,
e.g. ionisers, water filters, and where
they can be bought. Publishes a
newsletter every three months. Send
stamped, addressed envelope for
reply.

**The Asthma Society**
300 Upper Street, Islington, London
N1 2XX. Tel: 01–226 2260. Supplies
information about asthma, list of
books for sale and details of local
branches.

**Arthritis and Rheumatism Council**
41 Eagle Street, London WC1R
4AR. Tel: 01–405 8572. Publishes
magazine half yearly.

**Bio-Health Ltd**
13 Oakdale Road, London SW16
2HP. Tel: 01–769 7975. Manufactures additive-free vitamin and
mineral tablets.

**British Diabetic Association**
10 Queen Anne Street, London
W1M OBD. Tel: 01–323 1531.
Supplies general and dietary information for diabetics.

**British Goat Society**
Secretary: Mrs. T. May, Rougham,
Bury St Edmunds, Suffolk IP30 9LJ.
Tel: 0359 70351. Supplies list of local
affiliated societies who will inform
you of nearest goats' milk supplier.

**British Homoeopathic Association**
27A Devonshire Street, London
W1N 1RJ. Tel: 01–935 2163. Supplies information on homoeopathy,
list of doctors and hospitals
practising it in your area, and list of
pharmacies stocking homoeopathic
medicines.

**British Sheep Dairying Association**
Mrs Olivia Mills, Secretary, Wield
Wood, Alresford, Hampshire SO24
9RU. Tel: 0420 63151. Supplies list of
local sheep's milk suppliers and
shops selling their produce. Send
stamped, self-addressed envelope for
reply.

**British Society of Allergy and
Environmental Medicine**
Hon. Secretary, The Medical Centre,
Hythe, Southampton, SO4 5ZB. Tel:
0703 845955. Supplies list of doctors
specialising in allergies (although not
necessarily allergy to food).

**College of Health**
18 Victoria Park Square, London E2 9PF. Tel: 01–980 6263. Formed to encourage people to look after their own health, it publishes 'Self-Health' magazine every 3 months and organises local groups.

**Cry-sis**
63 Putney Road, Freezywater, Enfield, Middlesex, EN3 6NN. Tel: 027–978 371. Voluntary self-help group giving support and help to parents of babies who cry excessively. Organises local groups and publishes a newsletter every four months.

**Ecoropa Ltd**
Crickhowell, Powys, NP8 1TA, Wales. Ecological action group. Campaigns and issues leaflets promoting purer environment and food.

**FACT, Food Additives Campaign Team**
Room W, 25 Horsell Road, London N5 1XL. Campaigning for a tighter control of the use of food additives, more investigation into their effects on health and for more information to be made avaialable to the general public.

**Food Watch**
Butts Pond Ind. Estate, Sturminster Newton, DT10 1AZ. Tel: 0258 73356. Sells substitute foods for special diets.

**Friends of the Earth**
377 City Road, London EC1V 1NA. Tel: 01–837 0731.

**Henry Doubleday Research Association** Ryton Court, Ryton on Dunsmore, Coventry, CV8 3LG. Tel: Coventry 0203 303517. Publishes The Organic Food Guide price £2.50 + 50p p&p.

**Here's Health**
30 Station Approach, West Byfleet, Surrey KT14 6NF. Tel: 09323 49123. A monthly magazine.

**Hyperactive Children's Support Group** Secretary: Sally Bunday, 59 Meadowside, Angmering, West Sussex, BN16 4BW. Tel: Littlehampton 0903 725182 (mornings). Supplies information and advice on diet and how to deal with hyperactive children, details of local groups and publishes a magazine every 4 months. Send stamped, self-addressed envelope for reply.

**Irish Allergy Treatment and Research Association**
PO Box 1067, Churchtown, Dublin 14 Eire. Publishes journal.

**The London Food Commission**
PO Box 291, London N5 1DU. Tel: 01–633 5782. Provides independent information, education and advice on all aspects of food. Publishes a newsletter every 3 months.

**Migraine Trust**
45 Great Ormond Street, London WC1N 3HD. Tel: 01–278 2676. Publishes booklet 'Understanding Migraine' and sponsors Princess Margaret Migraine Clinic at London's Charing Cross Hospital.

**National Eczema Society**
Tavistock House North, Tavistock Square, London WC1H 9SR. Tel: 01–388 4097. Publishes information about eczema and how to cope with it including general advice on diet. Publishes newsletter every 3 months which is very informative and may be useful to allergy sufferers of other

symptoms. Provides details of local area groups.

**National Society for Research into Allergy** PO Box 45, Hinckley, Leicester, LE10 1JY. Tel: 0455 635212. Publishes elimination diet and food reintroduction booklet; journal called 'Reaction' every 3 months; list of allergy self-help groups; and will supply name of local allergy specialist. Send stamp addressed envelope for reply.

**New Health**
Haymarket Publishing Ltd, Subscriptions, 12–14 Ansdell Street, London W8 5TR. Tel: 01–937 7288. Editorial: 01–892 4460. A monthly magazine.

**Organic Farm Foods**
Unit 7, Allerslie Square, Lyham Road, London SW2. Tel: 01–274 0234. Will inform you of nearest shop or wholesaler.

**Society of Environmental Therapy**
521 Foxhall Road, Ipswich, Suffolk IP3 8LW. Tel: 0473 73552. Journal every 3 months.

**The Soil Association**
86 Colston Street, Bristol, BS1 5BB. Tel: 0272 290661. Allows farmers and growers of organically grown fruit and vegetables to use its trade mark symbol if their produce meets its set standards. A list of its symbol holders is available by post for £1.

# Appendix 2

# Additives: list of code numbers

These additives and their code numbers are used throughout the Common Market although some of them may be banned by individual member countries. They are also used in several other countries. In the UK either the code number or the actual name should be listed on labels as an ingredient. Some additives do not yet have code numbers and their full name should be shown. Missing numbers in this list refer to substances not allowed or not used. Some numbers are preceded by the letter E, others are not: this has no significance to the consumer. A few additives have more than one name and many carry out more than one function.

This list has been compiled from information supplied by Safeway Food Stores Ltd.

## Colourings

**E100**    **Curcumin** Orange yellow colour extracted from the spice turmeric for use in pastries.

**E101**    **Riboflavin, Lactoflavin, Vitamin $B_2$** Yellow orange colour, naturally occurring vitamin $B_2$ usually obtained from yeast or synthetically produced. Used to nutritionally enrich and fortify foods.

**101(a)**  **Riboflavin-5′-phosphate, Vitamin $B_2$** Derivative of E101.

**E102**    **Tartrazine, FD&C Yellow No 5** Widely used yellow orange colour in soft drinks, cakes, biscuits, puddings, desserts, meat products, sauces, tinned and convenience foods and confectionery. Azo dye (see p. 158).

E104    **Quinoline yellow** Greenish yellow dye often used with other yellow colours and found especially in smoked fish. Artificial colouring (see p. 159).

107    **Yellow 2G** Yellow azo dye used in similar products to E102 (see p. 158).

E110    **Sunset yellow FCF, Orange yellow S** Yellow colour frequently used with E102 and so appears in a similar range of products. Azo dye (see p. 158).

E120    **Cochineal, Carminic acid, Carmine of cochineal** Natural red colour obtained from egg yolk and dried insects but may be synthetically produced. Due to its high cost it is not frequently used.

E122    **Carmoisine, Azorubine** Red purple colour often added to raspberry and chocolate flavoured desserts, jam, cherryade, bottled sauce and breaded meat products. Azo dye (see p. 158).

E123    **Amaranth** Red colour sometimes used in gravy mix, jam and red coloured drinks. Azo dye (see p. 158).

E124    **Ponceau 4R, Cochineal red A, New cochine** Red colour used to restore the colour of tinned strawberries. Also added to strawberry jam, jelly and ice-cream, savoury rice, cheesecake mix and some meat products. Azo dye (see p. 158).

E127    **Erythrosine BS** Red colour rich in the mineral iodine. Used in glace-cherries, peach melba yogurt, vacuum packed ham and pork, tinned strawberries and certain crisp and potato snacks. Also may be used in plaque disclosing tablets and mouthwashes. Artificial colouring (see p. 159).

128    **Red 2G** Red colour providing the pink colour typically associated with pork pies, sausages and some other meat products. Azo dye (see p. 158).

E131    **Patent blue V** Artificial colouring (see p. 159).

E132    **Indigo carmine, Indigotine** Blue colouring added to gravy mix and certain meat products. Artificial colouring (see p. 159).

**E133**     **Brilliant blue FCF, FD&C Blue No 1** Blue colour often combined with E102 to produce green colour used in bacon flavour snacks. Artificial colouring (see p. 159).

**E140**     **Chlorophyll** Naturally occurring green pigment found in the leaves or stems of plants. Nature identical synthetically produced chlorophyll may be added to processed green vegetables to increase their colour.

**E141**     **Copper complexes of chlorophyll and chlorophyllins** Green colour obtained by a reaction between copper and nature identical synthetically produced chlorophyll. Used to heighten the green colour of products such as cucumber relish.

**E142**     **Green S, Acid brilliant green BS, Lissamine green** Restores the green colour to tinned peas. Also added to asparagus soup, lemon or lime drinks and jellies and mint sauce. Artificial colouring (see p. 159).

**E150**     **Caramel** Commonly used brown colour and flavouring (see Caramel p. 157).

**E151**     **Black PN, Brilliant black BN** Black colouring frequently used to darken fruity sauce. Azo dye (see p. 158).

**E153**     **Carbon black, Vegetable carbon** Natural or nature identical synthetically produced black colour obtained from burnt plant material.

**154**     **Brown FK** Brown colour often added to smoked fish especially kippers. Azo dye (see p. 158).

**155**     **Chocolate brown HT** Brown azo dye (see p. 158).

**E160**     **Carotenoids and their derivatives: E160(a)-(f)** Plant pigments occurring naturally in carrots, tomatoes, apricots, oranges, rosehips and green leafy vegetables, providing a range of natural colours from yellow to red. Their nature identical synthetically produced compounds are generally added to food.

**E160(a)**     **Alpha-carotene, Beta-carotene Gamma-carotene** Orange colour added to biscuits, cakes, margarine, creamed rice, cheese products and certain soups. Beta-carotene is a substance converted in the body to Vitamin A.

**E160(b)** **Annatto, Bixin, Norbixin** Orange peachy colour used in coffee creamer, pastry and some cheese and cheese products. (See Natural Food Colour p. 157).

**E160(c)** **Capsanthin, Capsorubin** Extracted from paprika. See E160.

**E160(d)** **Lycopene** See E160.

**E160(e)** **Beta-apo-8′-carotenal ($C_{30}$)** See E160.

**E160(f)** **Ethyl ester of beta-apo-8′-carotenoic acid ($C_{30}$)** See E160.

**E161** **Xanthrophylls: E161(a)-(i)** Carotenoid pigments providing natural yellow to red colours.

**E161(a)** **Flavoxanthin** See E161.

**E161(b)** **Lutein** See E161.

**E161(c)** **Cryptoxanthin** See E161.

**E161(d)** **Rubixanthin** See E161.

**E161(e)** **Violaxanthin** See E161.

**E161(f)** **Rhodoxanthin** See E161.

**E161(g)** **Canthaxanthin** See E161.

**E161(h)** **Zeaxanthin** Only used in poultry feed. See E161.

**E161(i)** **Citranaxanthin** Only used in poultry feed. See E161.

**E162** **Beetroot Red, Betanin** Natural red purple colour in beetroots which may be added to oxtail soup.

**E163** **Anthocyanins** Plant pigments with colours ranging from red to blue. Naturally present in red cabbage.

**E170** **Calcium carbonate, chalk** Naturally occurring mineral. Its various functions include acid regulator, firming agent, releasing agent and nutrient. It is added to white flour as a calcium supplement to replace the loss due to refining. Frequently an ingredient in bread and baked products.

**E171** **Titanium dioxide** Derived from a natural mineral.

**E172** **Iron oxides and hydroxides**

**E173** **Aluminium**

**E174** **Silver**

**E175** **Gold**

**E180** **Pigment rubine, Lithol rubine BK** Red azo dye (see p. 158).

- **Methyl violet** Not allowed in food but used to health stamp meat and mark citrus fruit.
- **Paprika**
- **Turmeric**
- **Saffron, Sandalwood**

## Preservatives and acids

E200    **Sorbic acid** Naturally occurs in some fruit but generally manufactured synthetically for use as a preservative. Often added to cottage cheese, cheese spread and frozen pizza.

E201    **Sodium sorbate** Derivative of sorbic acid (see E200).

E202    **Potassium sorbate** Often added to dried fruit eg prunes. Derivative of sorbic acid (see E200).

E203    **Calcium sorbate** Derivative of sorbic acid (see E200).

E210    **Benzoic acid** Naturally occurs in cherry bark, raspberries, tea, anise and cassia bark but is prepared synthetically for commercial food use. It functions as a preservative and antioxidant most frequently in fruit products and soft drinks but may also be found in pickles and salad dressings. See Benzoates p. 166.

E211    **Sodium benzoate** See Benzoates p. 166.

E212    **Potassium benzoate** See Benzoates p. 166.

E213    **Calcium benzoate** See Benzoates p. 166.

E214    **Ethyl para-hydroxybenzoate, Ethyl 4-hydroxybenzoate** See Benzoates p. 166.

E215    **Ethyl 4-hydroxybenzoate sodium salt** See Benzoates p. 166.

E216    **Propyl 4-hydroxybenzoate** See Benzoates p. 166.

E217    **Propyl 4-hydroxybenzoate sodium salt** See Benzoates p. 166.

E218    **Methyl 4-hydroxybenzoate** See Benzoates p. 166.

E219    **Methyl 4-hydroxybenzoate sodium salt** See Benzoates p. 166.

201 Appendix 2 Additives: list of code numbers

**E220**    **Sulphur dioxide** Gas prepared chemically for use in food as preservative, flour improver, bleaching agent and Vitamin C stabilizer. Often used in carbonated drinks, marmalade, glace cherries and mixed peel, cakes, fruit based products, dried fruit and meat products. See p. 167.

**E221**    **Sodium sulphite** Derivative of sulphur dioxide. See E220.

**E222**    **Sodium bisulphite, Sodium hydrogen sulphite** Synthetic preservative and bleaching agent often added to wine and beer. Derivative of sulphur dioxide. See E220.

**E223**    **Sodium metabisulphite** Synthetic preservative added to sausages and some bottled sauces and soft drinks. Derivative of sulphur dioxide. See E220.

**E224**    **Potassium metabisulphite** Derivative of E220.

**E226**    **Calcium sulphite** Derivative of sulphur dioxide. See E220.

**E227**    **Calcium bisulphite, Calcium hydrogen sulphite** Derivative of sulphur dioxide. See E220.

**E230**    **Diphenyl, Biphenyl**

**E231**    **Orthophenylphenol, 2-Hydroxybiphenyl**

**E232**    **Sodium orthophenylphenate, Sodium biphenyl-2-yl oxide**

**E233**    **Thiabendazole, 2-(Thiazol-4 yl) benzimidazole**

**234**     **Nisin**

**E239**    **Hexamine, Hexamethylenetetramine**

**E249**    **Potassium nitrite** Naturally occurring mineral used in cooked meats, sausages and cured meats as a preservative and a colour fixative. See Nitrates p. 167.

**E250**    **Sodium nitrite** Derived from sodium nitrate (E251) by chemical or bacterial action. Preservative and colour fixative in cured meats, creating the characteristic pink colour. Added to cooked and cured meats, bacon and pork sausages. See Nitrates p. 167.

**E251**    **Sodium nitrate** Naturally occurring mineral usually manufactured synthetically for food use as a preservative and colour fixative in cooked meats, bacon, ham and some cheese. See Nitrates p. 167.

**E252**   **Potassium nitrate** Occurs naturally but may be produced artificially from waste animal and vegetable material. This additive is one of the oldest and most effective preservatives for meat and also functions as a curing agent. However it may cause stomach irritation and an irregular pulse in susceptible individuals. See Nitrates p. 167.

**E260**   **Acetic acid** Natural component of vinegar but generally manufactured from wood for use as a food preservative, acid or colour dilutant. Typically added to pickles, bottled sauces and chutneys.

**E261**   **Potassium acetate** Derivative of E260.

**E262**   **Sodium hydrogen diacetate** Derivative of E260.

**262**    **Sodium acetate** Derivative of E260.

**E270**   **Lactic acid** Produced by the fermentation of lactose (the sugar present in milk). It occurs naturally in soured milk and yogurt. It acts as an acid, a preservative and a flavour and assists the action of antioxidants. Widely used additive to be found in margarine, infant milks, pickled red cabbage, cheese spread, salad dressings, cakes, biscuits, confectionery and some prepared meat dishes.

**E280**   **Propionic acid** Fatty acid produced by animals during their digestion process but also manufactured synthetically for food application. Functions as a preservative when added to baked foods and dairy products. See p. 167.

**E281**   **Sodium propionate** Derivative of E280.

**E282**   **Calcium propionate** Derivative of E280.

**E283**   **Potassium propionate** Derivative of E280.

**E290**   **Carbon dioxide** Gas present in air but produced synthetically to carbonate fizzy drinks. It also acts as a coolant, freezant, propellant, preservative and packaging gas.

# Miscellaneous

| | |
|---|---|
| **296** | **Malic acid (DL or L)** |
| **297** | **Fumaric acid** Occurs naturally but prepared synthetically for use as an acid flavour. Added to baked products and cheese cake mix. |
| **-** | **DL-Tartaric acid** |
| **-** | **Monosodium DL-tartrate** |
| **-** | **Disodium DL-tartrate** |
| **-** | **Monopotassium DL-tartrate** |
| **-** | **Dipotassium DL-tartrate** |
| **-** | **Potassium sodium DL-tartrate** |

# Antioxidants

| | |
|---|---|
| **E300** | **L-Ascorbic acid, Vitamin C** Occurs naturally in fruit and vegetables and is also synthesised biologically. Besides being a nutrient, it acts as a preservative, antioxidant, meat colour fixative and flour improver. It is often added to mashed potato, fruit juices, bread and baked products. |
| **E301** | **Sodium L-Ascorbate, Vitamin C** Derivative of E300. Often added to cured meats. |
| **E302** | **Calcium L-Ascorbate, Vitamin C** Derivative of E300. |
| **E304** | **Ascorbyl palmitate, 6-0-Palmitoyl-L-ascorbic acid** Derivative of E300. |
| **E306** | **Extracts of natural origin rich in tocopherols, Vitamin E** Obtained from soya bean oil, wheatgerm, rice germ, cottonseed, maize and green leaves. Added to some fats and oils as an antioxidant and nutrient. |
| **E307** | **Synthetic alpha-tocopherol, Vitamin E** Added to fats and oils as an antioxidant and nutrient. |
| **E308** | **Synthetic gamma-tocopherol, Vitamin E** Added to fats and oils as an antioxidant and nutrient. |
| **E309** | **Synthetic delta-tocopherol, Vitamin E** Added to fats and oils as an antioxidant and nutrient. |
| **E310** | **Propyl gallate** Synthetically prepared antioxidant added to fats and oils. Exists in some fried foods. It may impart a bitter taste. See Gallates p. 168. |

E311        **Octyl gallate** Synthetically prepared antioxidant added to
fats and oils. Exists in some fried foods. It may impart a
bitter taste. See Gallates p. 168.

E312        **Dodecyl gallate** Synthetically prepared antioxidant added
to fats and oils. Exists in some fried foods. It may impart a
bitter taste. See Gallates p. 168.

E320        **Butylated hydroxyanisole (BHA)** Antioxidant manufactured synthetically for use alone or in conjunction with
E310, E280 or E330. Often found in crisps and potato
snacks, biscuits, pastry, bottled sauces and fried foods (see
p. 168).

E321        **Butylated hydroxytoluene (BHT)** Synthetically prepared
antioxidant. Usage is very similar to that of E320 (see p.
168).

## Miscellaneous (continued)

E322        **Lecithins** Type of fat or liquid compound found naturally
in all living organisms. Protective against cholesterol
deposition in the body. Egg yolk is a very rich source but
for commercial use it is usually obtained from soya beans.
Used as an antioxidant and emulsifier in chocolate and
chocolate products, powdered milk, margarine and potato
snacks.

E325        **Sodium lactate** Humectant added to cheese and confectionery to keep food moist. Salt of lactic acid (see E270).

E326        **Potassium lactate** Acidity regulator. Salt of lactic acid (see
E270).

E327        **Calcium lactate** Acidity regulator and firming agent frequently used in baking powder. Salt of lactic acid (see
E270).

E330        **Citric acid** Occurs naturally in citrus fruits but may also be
prepared from the fermentation of molasses. It is often
added to soft drinks, pickles, bottled sauces, jams, dairy
and baked products where it functions as an antioxidant,
preservative, acid regulator and flour improver.

E331     **Sodium citrate, Monosodium citrate, Sodium dihydrogen citrate. Disodium citrate, Trisodium citrate** Salt of citric acid performing similar functions (see E330).

E332     **Potassium citrate, Monopotassium citrate, Potassium dihydrogen citrate, Tripotassium citrate** Salt of citric acid performing similar functions (see E331).

E333     **Calcium citrate, Monocalcium citrate, Dicalcium citrate, Tricalcium citrate** Acts as an acidity regulator, emulsifier and firming agent and may be found in carbonated drinks, wines, confectionery and cheese products. Salt of citric acid (see E330).

E334     **Tartaric acid, L-tartaric acid** Natural product of wine making added to baking powder as an acidity regulator.

E335     **Sodium tartrate, Monosodium tartrate, Disodium tartrate** Salt of tartaric acid performing similar functions (see E334).

E336     **Cream of tartar, Monopotassium tartrate, Dipotassium tartrate, Potassium tartrate, Potassium hydrogen tartrate** A well-known ingredient of baking powder. Salt of tartaric acid (see E334).

E337     **Potassium sodium tartrate** Salt of tartaric acid (see E334).

E338     **Phosphoric acid, Orthophosphoric acid**

E339     **Sodium dihydrogen orthophosphate, Disodium hydrogen orthophosphate, Trisodium orthophosphate**

E340     **Potassium dihydrogen orthophosphate, Dipotassium hydrogen orthophosphate, Tripotassium orthophosphate**

E341     **Calcium tetrahydrogen diorthophosphate, Calcium hydrogen orthophosphate, Tricalcium diorthophosphate** Synthetic product of a naturally occurring mineral. Its functions include anti-caking agent, acidity regulator, emulsifier, flour improver, nutrient and aid to the action of antioxidants. Most likely to be found in potato snacks, pastry mix and baking powder.

350     **Sodium malate, Sodium hydrogen malate**

351     **Potassium malate**

352     **Calcium malate, Calcium hydrogen malate**

353     **Metatartaric acid**

| | |
|---|---|
| **355** | **Adipic acid** |
| **363** | **Succinic acid** |
| **370** | **1,-4-Heptono lactone** |
| **-** | **Calcium heptonate** |
| **-** | **Sodium heptonate** |
| **375** | **Nicotinic acid, Vitamin B₃** B group vitamin naturally occurring in meat, fish, cereals and vegetables. Can be synthetically produced and is added to certain breakfast cereals and white flour. |
| **-** | **Tannic acid** |
| **380** | **Triammonium citrate** |
| **381** | **Ammonium ferric citrate** |
| **385** | **Calcium disodium EDTA, Calcium disodium ethylenediamine-NNN 'N' tetra-acetate** |
| **-** | **Disodium dihydrogen EDTA** |
| **-** | **Ethoxyquin** |
| **-** | **Diphenylamine** |

## Emulsifiers, stabilisers and miscellaneous additives

| | |
|---|---|
| **E400** | **Alginic acid** Emulsifier, stabiliser, gelling agent or thickener extracted from brown seaweed. Frequently added to ice cream, instant desserts and puddings. |
| **E401** | **Sodium alginate** Derivative of E400. |
| **E402** | **Potassium alginate** Derivative of E400. |
| **E403** | **Ammonium alginate** Derivative of E400. |
| **E404** | **Calcium alginate** Derivative of E400. |
| **E405** | **Propylene glycol alginate, Propane-1, 2-diol alginate** Derivative of E400. |
| **E406** | **Agar** Naturally occurring gum extracted from seaweeds and related marine plants which is not digested and therefore acts as a source of dietary fibre. Is a stabiliser and gelling agent in the jelly surrounding tinned ham and in meat glazes. |
| **E407** | **Carrageenan, Irish moss** Gum naturally present in red seaweed which provides a source of fibre. Acts as an emulsifier, stabiliser and gelling agent. Most commonly used in ice cream, also found in salad dressings. |

**E408**  **Furcellaran**

**E410**  **Carob gum, Locust bean gum** Natural extract from the carob tree seed. Provides a source of fibre. Acts as an emulsifier, stabiliser and gelling agent. Added to ice cream and certain soups. Carob is a non-caffeine substitute for cocoa and chocolate (see p. 136).

**E412**  **Guar gum, Cluster bean gum** Naturally occurring seed gum from a tree of the pea family, used as a stabiliser and thickener. Has been tested in diabetic foods because its fibrous nature reduces the rate of absorption of other food components with which it is combined, such as sugar. Added to cottage cheese, bottled sauces, soup, ice cream and frozen desserts.

**E413**  **Tragacanth** Natural gum obtained from a tree of the pea family. Acts as an emulsifier, stabiliser and thickener. May be used to prevent the crystallisation of sugar in confectionery.

**E414**  **Gum arabic, Acacia** Origin and uses very similar to E413.

**E415**  **Xanthan gum** Prepared by fermenting a carbohydrate with a bacteria. Acts as an emulsifier, stabiliser and thickener. Frequently added to ice cream, cottage cheese and bottled sauces.

**416**  **Karaya gum**

**E420**  **Sorbitol, Sorbitol syrup** A sweetener. Occurs naturally in certain berries and fruit but is generally produced from glucose which is derived from corn (maize). Taken in large quantities may have a laxative effect. Widely used in diabetic confectionery, preserves, biscuits, cakes, soft drinks and toothpaste. Also acts as a humectant and food colour dilutant.

**E421**  **Mannitol** A sweetener derived from mannose but generally prepared for commercial use from seaweed. Used in confectionery, ice cream and desserts. Also acts as an emulsifier, anti-caking agent and thickener.

**E422**  **Glycerol** Naturally present in many plants but prepared commercially from fats and oils for use as a humectant in liqueurs, confectionery and cake icing.

| | |
|---|---|
| 430 | **Polyoxyethylene (8) stearate** |
| 431 | **Polyoxyethylene (40) stearate** |
| 432 | **Polysorbate 20** Derivative of sorbitol (E420). |
| 433 | **Polysorbate 80** Derivative of sorbitol (E420). |
| 434 | **Polysorbate 40** Derivative of sorbitol (E420). |
| 435 | **Polysorbate 60** Derivative of sorbitol (E420). Functions as an emulsifier and stabiliser. Frequently added to bread and baked products. |
| 436 | **Polysorbate 65** Derivative of sorbitol (E420). |
| E440(a) | **Pectin** Occurs naturally in fruits, roots and stems of plants. Used as a stabiliser and gelling agent in preserves, jellies and mint jelly. |
| E440(b) | **Amidated pectin** Chemically treated pectin added to preserves and jellies as an emulsifier and gelling agent. |
| 442 | **Ammonium phosphatides** |
| E450(a) | **Disodium dihydrogen diphosphate, Trisodium diphosphate, Tetrasodium diphosphate, Tetrapotassium diphosphate** Synthetically prepared emulsifiers and stabilisers. Sometimes used to retain moisture in meat products, especially frozen poultry. Used in bread, sausages, meat (in particular cured and canned meats) and fish products, cheese spread and cheese products. |
| E450(b) | **Pentasodium triphosphate, Pentapotassium triphosphate** Similar to E450(a). |
| E450(c) | **Sodium polyphosphates, Potassium polyphosphates** Similar to E450(a). |
| E460 | **Powdered cellulose, Microcrystalline cellulose, Alphacellulose** Fibrous part of plants. Indigestible and therefore a bulking agent providing fibre. Also acts as an emulsifier, stabiliser, anti-caking agent and thickener. May be used in high fibre bread and low calorie products. |
| E461 | **Methylcellulose** Widely used in slimming tablets and formulas to create a feeling of fullness without extra calories. It does this by absorbing water and swelling in the stomach. Derivative of E460. |

E463    **Hydroxypropylcellulose** Derivative of E460 performing similar functions.

E464    **Hydroxypropylmethylcellulose** Derivative of E460 performing similar functions.

E465    **Ethylmethylcellulose** May be added to cakes. Derivative of E460 performing similar functions.

E466    **Carboxymethylcellulose sodium salt (CMC)** May be used in some dairy products and cheesecake mix. Derivative of E460 performing similar functions.

E470    **Sodium, potassium and calcium salts of fatty acids** Synthetically produced emulsifiers, stabilisers and anti-caking agents found in crisps and potato snacks.

E471    **Mono- and di-glycerides of fatty acids** Main constituents of animal and vegetable fats and oils. Normal products of fat but are prepared synthetically for commercial use. Frequently added to packet soup, cake, crisps and potato snacks, bread and baked products and margarine.

E472(a)    **Acetic acid esters of mono- and di-glycerides of fatty acids** Emulsifier, stabiliser, thickener, humectant, releasing agent. Used in soups, bread and baked products, cheesecake mix. Derivative of E471.

E472(b)    **Lactoglycerides, lactic acid esters of mono- and di-glycerides of fatty acids** Similar uses and functions as E472(a).

E472(c)    **Citroglycerides, Citric acid esters of mono- and di-glycerides of fatty acids** Similar uses and functions as E472(a).

E472(d)    **Tartaric acid esters of mono- and di-glycerides of fatty acids** Similar uses and functions as E472(a).

E472(e)    **Mono- and di-acetyltartaric acid esters of mono- and di-glycerides of fatty acids** Similar uses and functions as E472(a).

E473    **Sucrose esters of fatty acids**

E474    **Sucroglycerides**

E475     **Polyglycerol esters of fatty acids** Used as an emulsifier and stabiliser in puddings and packet cheesecakes. Synthetic product of E471.

476     **Polyglycerol polyricinoleate, Polyglycerol esters of poly-condensed fatty acids of castor oil**

E477     **Propane-1,2-diol esters of fatty acids**

478     **Lactylated fatty acid esters of glycerol and propane-1,2-diol**

E481     **Sodium stearoyl-2-lactylate** Prepared synthetically from lactic acid (E270). A stabiliser and emulsifier used in crisps and potato snacks.

E482     **Calcium stearoyl-2-lactylate** Prepared synthetically from lactic acid (E270). A stabiliser and emulsifier used in crisps and potato snacks.

E483     **Stearyl tartrate**

491     **Sorbitan monostearate** Synthetically produced for use as a stabiliser, glazing agent and emulsifier in cakes, cake mixes, whipped dessert toppings and other baked goods.

492     **Sorbitan tristearate**

493     **Sorbitan monolaurate**

494     **Sorbitan mono-oleate**

495     **Sorbitan monopalmitate**

\-     **Pectin extract**

\-     **Polyglycerol esters of dimerised fatty acids of soya bean oil**

\-     **Oxidatively thermally polymerised soya bean oil interacted with mono- and di-glycerides**

\-     **Dioctyl sodium sulphosuccinate**

\-     **Extract of quillaia**

\-     **Sodium stearate**

\-     **Potassium stearate**

\-     **Calcium stearate**

\-     **Butyl stearate**

500     **Bicarbonate of soda, Sodium carbonate, Sodium hydrogen carbonate** Prepared synthetically for use as an acid regulator, firming agent, release agent, raising agent and dilutant. Often added to malted drinks, tinned custard, cheesy potato snacks, bread and bread products.

501     **Potassium carbonate, Potassium hydrogen carbonate**
503     **Ammonium carbonate, Ammonium hydrogen carbonate**
504     **Magnesium carbonate** Naturally occurring mineral functioning as an acid regulator in sour cream, butter and ice cream and an anti-caking agent in table salt and icing sugar.
507     **Hydrochloric acid**
508     **Potassium chloride** Present naturally, often associated with rock salt. Used as an emulsifier, stabiliser, salt substitute and dietary supplement. Similar taste to table salt. Found in low sodium or low salt products.

509     **Calcium chloride, Calcium chloride anhydrous** Product of natural salt brine which may be prepared chemically. Added to red kidney beans to act as a firming agent and prevent texture deterioration.

510     **Ammonium chloride**
513     **Sulphuric acid**
514     **Sodium sulphate**
515     **Potassium sulphate**
516     **Calcium sulphate**
518     **Magnesium sulphate**
-       **Ammonium sulphate**
-       **Aluminium potassium sulphate**
-       **Potassium persulphate**
-       **Ammonium persulphate**
524     **Sodium hydroxide**
525     **Potassium hydroxide**
526     **Calcium hydroxide**
527     **Ammonium hydroxide**
528     **Magnesium hydroxide**
529     **Calcium oxide**
530     **Magnesium oxide, heavy and light**
535     **Sodium ferrocyanide, Sodium hexacyanoferrate II**
536     **Potassium ferrocyanide, Potassium hexacyanoferrate II**
540     **Dicalcium diphosphate**

541   **Sodium aluminium phosphate acidic and basic** Synthetically prepared raising agent functional in self-raising flour and therefore will appear in many baked products.

542   **Edible bone phosphate** Mineral supplement and anticaking agent extracted from animal bones. Also used as a filler for tablets.

544   **Calcium polyphosphates**

545   **Ammonium polyphosphates**

-     **Ammonium dihydrogen orthophosphate**

-     **Diammonium hydrogen orthophosphate**

551   **Silicon dioxide, Silica** Derived from sand or rock and processed for use in shaped crisps as an anti-caking agent.

552   **Calcium silicate** Salt of silicon dioxide (551) performing similar functions. Also a glazing agent, acid regulator, releasing agent and a coating agent in chewing gum and some rice grains to prevent sticking. Also found in meat pies, salt and confectionery.

553(a) **Magnesium silicate synthetic, Magnesium trisilicate**

553(b) **Talc**

554   **Sodium aluminium silicate** Frequently added to packet noodles.

556   **Calcium aluminium silicate**

558   **Bentonite**

559   **Kaolin**

570   **Stearic acid**

572   **Magnesium stearate**

575   **Glucono delta lactone, D-Glucono-1,5-lactone**

576   **Sodium gluconate**

577   **Potassium gluconate**

578   **Calcium gluconate**

# Gases

- Nitrous oxide
- Nitrogen
- Hydrogen
- Oxygen
- Octadecylammonium acetate
- Oxystearin
- Polydextrose
- Calcium phytate
- Dichlorodifluoremethane
- 2-Aminoethanol

# Flavour enhancers

620   **L-Glutamic acid** See p. 162.

621   **Monosodium glutamate, MSG, Sodium hydrogen L-glutamate** Naturally present in seaweed but more frequently prepared from sugar beet. See p. 162 for more details.

622   **Monopotassium glutamate, Potassium hydrogen L-glutamate** See p. 162.

623   **Calcium glutamate, Calcium dihydrogen di-L-glutamate** See p. 162.

627   **Sodium guanylate, Guanosine 5′-disodium phosphate** Occurs naturally in sardines and yeast extract but manufactured synthetically for use as a flavour enhancer. Often added to crisps and potato snacks, gravy granules and pre-cooked dried rice. Best avoided by people suffering from gout.

631   **Sodium inosinate, Inosine 5′-disodium phosphate** May be prepared from sardines and meat extract. Similar to 627.

635   **Sodium 5′-ribonucleotide** Mixture of 627 and 631 most frequently added to crisps, packet soups and potato products.

636   **Maltol**

637   **Ethyl Maltol**

## Glazing agents

900      **Dimethylpolysiloxane** Also an anti-foaming agent.
901      **Beeswax, white and yellow**
903      **Carnauba wax**
904      **Shellac**
905      **Mineral hydrocarbons, paraffins**
907      **Refined microcrystallin wax**
—      **Sperm oil**
—      **Spermaceti**
—      **Glycine**

## Bleaching agents and flour improvers

920      **L-cysteine hydrochloride (anhydrous and monohydrate)** See Bread p. 124.

924      **Potassium bromate** Oxidising agent, flour improver and bleaching agent manufactured synthetically for use in flour and thus bread and baked products. It may cause nausea, abdominal pain and diarrhoea in susceptible individuals and, as a result of the bleaching properties, cause loss of vitamin E from the flour. See Bread p. 124.

925      **Chlorine** Synthetically prepared bleaching agent used in flour. Causes loss of vitamin E and may cause irritation in some people. Found in white flour, white bread cakes and puddings. See White Flour p. 123.

926      **Chlorine dioxide** Synthetically prepared additive with properties and uses as Chlorine (925). It also acts as a water purifier, bleaching agent and oxidising agent. It is used in white flour. See White Flour p. 123.

927      **Azoformamide, Azodicarbonamide** Chemically manufactured flour improver used to increase the dough tolerance to various fermentation conditions brought about by yeast action. A common ingredient in flour, bread and baked products. See Bread p. 124.

—      **Benzoyl peroxide** Bleaching agent. See Benzoates p. 166 and White Flour p. 123.

# Sweeteners

- **Saccharin** Non-nutritive, calorie free, artificial sweetener with a bitter after taste. Used as a source of sweetening in low calorie products and often appears in addition to sugar in soft drinks and confectionery. See p. 169.
- **Calcium saccharin** (see saccharin above).
- **Sodium saccharin** (see saccharin above).
- **Acesulfame potassium**
- **Aspartame** New artificial sweetener of protein origin providing negligible calories. Contains the amino acid phenylalanine (PHE) so should be avoided by children with phenylketonuria (inborn error of metabolism). Sweetening agent in 'Candarel' and 'Nutra Sweet' products. Found in confectionery, low calorie desserts and soft drinks.
- **Thaumatin**
- **Hydrogenated glucose syrup**
- **Isomalt**
- **Xylitol**

# Appendix 3

# Main foods which caused allergy

| Allergy | Letters received[1] | Cows' milk[2] | Wheat | Eggs | Veg. | Nuts | Yeast | Fish |
|---|---|---|---|---|---|---|---|---|
| **Breathing** Asthma, hayfever, cold-like symptoms | 61 | 22 | 11 | 5 | 3 | 4 | 4 | 1 |
| **Skin** Eczema, rashes and swellings | 73 | 26 | 13 | 19 | 7 | 4 | — | 4 |
| **Headaches and migraine** | 29 | 10 | 4 | 4 | 3 | 1 | 2 | — |
| **Hyperactivity in children** | 28 | 6 | 2 | 2 | 1 | — | — | — |
| **Bedwetting and lack of bladder control** | 6 | — | 1 | — | — | — | — | — |
| **Stomach** Indigestion, cramps, sickness, diarrhoea | 19 | 5 | 6 | 1 | 1 | 1 | — | 1 |
| **Depression and nightmares in adults** | 3 | — | 2 | 1 | — | — | — | — |
| **Aches, pains and arthritis** | 6 | 1 | 2 | 1 | — | 1 | — | — |
| **Fits and convulsions** | 2 | 2 | — | — | — | — | — | — |
| **Shaking or fainting** | 3 | — | — | — | — | — | — | — |

1 Some people had symptoms from more than one food. Usually only certain foods within each category caused symptoms. 2 Includes cheese. 3 Monosodium glutamate.

| Meat | Fruit | Choc-olate | Coffee | Sugar | MSG³ | Preser-vative | Colour | Allergy |
|---|---|---|---|---|---|---|---|---|
| 3 | 2 | 5 | 2 | 7 | 5 | 6 | 18 | **Breathing** Asthma, hayfever, cold-like symptoms |
| 5 | 15 | 4 | 2 | 2 | 5 | 6 | 24 | **Skin** Eczema, rashes and swellings |
| 1 | 2 | 13 | 8 | 1 | 6 | 2 | 2 | **Headaches and migraine** |
| — | 4 | 4 | 1 | 2 | 2 | 9 | 17 | **Hyperactivity in children** |
| — | 2 | — | — | 1 | 1 | 4 | 4 | **Bedwetting and lack of bladder control** |
| 1 | 4 | 1 | 1 | 2 | — | 2 | 4 | **Stomach** Indigestion, cramps, sickness, diarrhoea |
| 1 | — | 1 | — | — | 1 | — | — | **Depression and nightmares in adults** |
| — | 2 | 1 | 2 | — | 1 | — | 1 | **Aches, pains and arthritis** |
| — | — | — | — | — | — | — | 1 | **Fits and convulsions** |
| — | — | — | — | — | 3 | — | — | **Shaking or fainting** |

# Index

# ORDER FORM

## EXTRA COPIES OF BOOK

If a friend wants to borrow your copy of ALLERGY? THINK ABOUT FOOD why not suggest they get their own? Or you may want to give one to someone you know. Further copies are available at £2.95 plus 40p p&p (UK) or £5 airmail (US $8).

Order your charts (see overleaf) and/or additional copies of the book by using the order form below which can be cut without harming your copy. Or if you prefer write a letter with your order instead, including your cheque or postal order to Wisebuy Publications, PO Box 379, London NW3 1NJ.

---

To: **Wisebuy Publications, PO Box 379, London NW3 1NJ**

Please send me _____ sets of 12 ALLERGY? THINK ABOUT FOOD CHARTS at £1.95 per set plus 40p p&p or £4 airmail (US $7).

Please send me _____ copies of ALLERGY? THINK ABOUT FOOD at £2.95 per copy plus 40p p&p or £5 airmail (US $8).

I enclose cheque/PO for £_____ payable to Wisebuy Publications

*Block letters please*

Name_____

Address_____

_____

_____ Post code_____

# ALLERGY? *THINK ABOUT FOOD* CHART

THIS SHEET can help you relate your symptoms to the cause. You can chart different foods as well as other possible causes e.g. weather conditions, pollen count, exposure to fumes.

● Use one sheet for each month, write in the current month and year e.g. March 1985.
● Fill in the days of the week before you start e.g. M for Monday.
● Note details of symptoms and everything you eat separately in two pocket diaries. Once or twice a month transfer details from the diaries to the chart.
● Symptoms can appear up to 24 hours later, maybe even longer, after eating a food. They may last up to four days, possibly longer.
● Try cutting out foods you suspect and see if the pattern alters.

*This chart is based on the system explained in the book 'Allergy? Think About Food' published by Wisebuy Publications, PO Box 379, London NW3 1NJ, price £2.95 plus 30p p & p.*

| FOOD | 1 | 2 | 3 | 4 | 5 | 6 | 7 | 8 | 9 | 10 | 11 | 12 | 13 | 14 | 15 | 16 | 17 | 18 | 19 | 20 | 21 | 22 | 23 | 24 | 25 | 26 | 27 | 28 | 29 | 30 | 31 |
|---|---|---|---|---|---|---|---|---|---|---|---|---|---|---|---|---|---|---|---|---|---|---|---|---|---|---|---|---|---|---|---|
| | | | | | | | | | | | | | | | | | | | | | | | | | | | | | | | |

| SYMPTOM OR MEDICINE CHART | If Medicine taken | | | | | | | | | | | | | | | | | | | | | | | | | | | | | | | |
|---|---|---|---|---|---|---|---|---|---|---|---|---|---|---|---|---|---|---|---|---|---|---|---|---|---|---|---|---|---|---|---|---|
| | 6 DOSES | | | | | | | | | | | | | | | | | | | | | | | | | | | | | | | |
| | 5 DOSES | | | | | | | | | | | | | | | | | | | | | | | | | | | | | | | |
| If no Medicine taken | 4 DOSES | | | | | | | | | | | | | | | | | | | | | | | | | | | | | | | |
| | 3 DOSES | | | | | | | | | | | | | | | | | | | | | | | | | | | | | | | |
| TERRIBLE | 2 DOSES | | | | | | | | | | | | | | | | | | | | | | | | | | | | | | | |
| BAD | 1 DOSE | | | | | | | | | | | | | | | | | | | | | | | | | | | | | | | |
| SLIGHT | SLIGHT | | | | | | | | | | | | | | | | | | | | | | | | | | | | | | | |
| Month | Year | 1 | 2 | 3 | 4 | 5 | 6 | 7 | 8 | 9 | 10 | 11 | 12 | 13 | 14 | 15 | 16 | 17 | 18 | 19 | 20 | 21 | 22 | 23 | 24 | 25 | 26 | 27 | 28 | 29 | 30 | 31 |
| Fill in day, e.g. M. Tu. W. Th. F. Sa. Su. | | | | | | | | | | | | | | | | | | | | | | | | | | | | | | | | |

## FOOD CHART

A simple way to chart your or your child's allergy is to use the specially designed ALLERGY? THINK ABOUT FOOD CHART. How to use it is described in Chapter 3. A set of 12 charts (A4 size 12 in. × 8¼ in.) is available at £1.95 plus 40p p & p. See overleaf.